One Day at a Time

A Journey Through Pediatric Cancer

Published by Bell Asteri Publishing & Enterprises, LLC
209 West 2nd Street #177
Fort Worth TX 76102
www.bellasteri.com

Published in the United States of America

ISBN: 978-1-957604-37-4 (hardback)
ISBN: 978-1-957604-38-1 (paperback)
ISBN: 978-1-957604-39-8 (electronic book)

To PapPaw: Thanks for always being my
biggest supporter. We miss you!

"One day at a time" has been our mantra since the start of this grueling, cruel, and sometimes beautiful and inspiring journey.

PREFACE

Writing a book has been a long-time goal of mine since childhood. In junior high, I started writing for the local newspaper. I was one of a select few local students chosen for employment with the paper, writing weekly articles in a dedicated student section. After I completed my first article and saw my words jump out from the paper in my hand, I was hooked. I continued to write in college, graduate school, and in my professional life. Putting words on a page that describe my situation is cathartic, therapeutic, and beautiful. Sharing a story so powerful is an honor and a privilege I do not take lightly.

Being a writer is something that flows through my blood. A traumatic experience like childhood cancer allowed me to share our story, our words of encouragement, our frustrations, and our experience to promote change and advocate for others along the journey. Cole and I dove into our words, thoughts, feelings, and emotions and let them come to life. The writing process was cathartic for both of us and healing in a way. The ability to take a traumatic experience and describe what occurred in our lives in one particularly difficult time period allowed us to come to terms with the event and take away its power. Realizing we were not in control or responsible for a childhood cancer diagnosis is freeing and gives the control back to us by coming to terms with the journey on our own terms. I am beyond honored to share this accomplishment with my co-author, son, and inspiration for the book, Cole.

Experiencing a childhood cancer diagnosis is painful for everyone involved. We experienced many situations unique to our journey and decided to share our story in the hopes of making it easier for anyone who follows a similar path. "One day at a time" is all you need to remember. Those five words helped us in the deep, down, and dark moments and allowed us to focus on the present task at hand, not looking back and not looking forward, just focusing on that moment knowing that it will pass and our situation will change as the journey evolves. So, remember our words, our mantra, and our inspiration and take everything "one day at a time" and know you are not alone because we are right by your side, every step of the way.

If you are reading this book because you or someone you know is in a similar situation, please know that we are with you. Please take our words, our experience, our trauma and our triumph and let them comfort you, inspire you, and fuel your desire to join us in the biggest battle we have endured.

Even if you are not personally affected by cancer, we encourage you to fight with us because cancer is awful but pediatric cancer is downright terrible and our children deserve better. By sharing our trauma and the experience of pediatric cancer, we can encourage others to bind together and fight, advocate, and pressure to make change happen. Combining both a mom and son's experience shares a parent and child perspective of childhood cancer which is absolutely necessary to elicit the change needed.

Sharing the unique struggle of a teen undergoing cancer treatment who not only endures physical and mental trauma at a pivotal part of development, but who also doesn't quite fit into either the pediatric or adult oncology worlds, is an important step in making change, adding more resources for teens and young adults, and changing the approach to this unique population.

Join us in our battle whether you are fighting your own battle, know someone who is, or want to be inspired to make change happen. An army of the strongest, most courageous, and brave fighters, along with their caregivers, can and will conquer pediatric cancer, one day, one battle, and one triumph at a time.

CHAPTER 1

The Fight Isn't Over at the Sound of the Bell

Ringing the bell at the end of treatment for pediatric cancer is a miraculous symbol of completing one of the most arduous, dark, and downright difficult journeys a child can face. The bell, however, does not erase the experience of a childhood cancer journey nor does it throw the trauma into the abyss for it never to touch your soul again. Instead, ringing the bell takes the trauma and sets it on fire. The flame burns for all pediatric cancer families and fuels an unending need to advocate and fight for all.

Laura

Where did the idea of a bell ringing ceremony at the end of a round of poison filled IVs, injections, and pills originate? Perhaps it came from a boxing ring and the bell that dings, signifying the end of a round in the fight, or a bell that sounds in a school at the end of class. Whatever the purpose or idea behind the bell, I did learn that the University of Texas MD Anderson Cancer Center is credited with pioneering this celebration in the 1990s by U.S. Navy rear admiral Irve Le Moyne who replicated ringing the bell at the end of his treatment to honor the Navy tradition of bell ringing at the completion of a job or task.

Admiral Le Moyne took experiences from his day-to-day life in the Navy and applied them to the end of his cancer treatment. The Navy can certainly be a difficult position to occupy and I'm sure the tasks required of a sailor are no picnic. The same can be said of a cancer journey. A cancer warrior needs to endure procedures, medications, surgeries, hospital stays, and other unpleasant tasks that are extremely difficult to say the least. Remember, our story focuses on pediatric cancer with the warriors being children. This population is certainly too young to serve in the military and many are even too young to obtain their first job.

I say this to bring a face to your mind when describing our population and to conceptualize the absolute horror and trauma our children are facing. The battle these tiny (and not so tiny, in the case of Cole and his fellow teenage and AYA warriors) face is mind-numbing. As a parent, I would do anything to protect my children. But, the horrible fact is I could do nothing against the biggest threat Cole faced over the past three years.

With our children now in the front of your mind, I return to Admiral LeMoyne. I never met this warrior and only read of his experience during my research of the symbol of the bell and the entire ceremony my son recently had the honor of completing. Even without meeting this hero in person, I have an inkling of what he endured during his military service (my husband, father and grandfathers are all veterans) and his cancer journey (my son, father, and stepfather are all cancer warriors). I want to think that the admiral felt a sense of pride and accomplishment while ringing the bell as a sailor and knowing that amazing feeling, he wanted to replicate it at the end of his arduous cancer journey.

I don't know if Admiral LeMoyne knew how this tradition would spread like wildfire to almost every cancer clinic throughout the United States and even internationally, but I hope he was able to see the effect his celebration had on countless patients throughout the world since the 1990s and will no doubt continue for the foreseeable future.

I'll be honest - I had no idea where the concept of a bell ringing ceremony originated before writing this page. I did think its origins began on the boxing mat somewhere ringside waiting for a round of the fight to be finished. I was interested to learn the details regarding the Navy tradition of bell ringing when they were finished with a task because I did not know that long-standing tradition existed. My mind begins to wander and analyze the tradition even further speculating that maybe the Navy inspired the bell at the end of a boxing round, creating a domino effect of a tradition with deep roots of historical events leading to a ritual signifying the end of a journey.

The Navy, boxers, and schools all use this symbol to indicate the end of something. Even some factories and other places of employment use a bell to signal to their employees it is time for a break or the end of a shift. I wonder how many other groups or individuals use a metal clang or buzzing sound to signify something is done or finished.

Now that I think of it, in the movies and on television I've seen a mom or other character in the kitchen ringing the dinner bell as a signal to hungry children or family members. The clang signifies the end of cooking and the beginning of break time to come into the kitchen from wherever the family was roaming to sit together and eat.

Wherever the origins of this celebration lie, I do know this symbolic ceremony means the world to many cancer patients and their families. Ringing the bell is part of the ultimate goal when starting treatment. Taking the last statement into consideration signifies the difficulty of the journey. The fact that the end is the ultimate goal indicates the unpleasant nature of the cancer experience, further glorifying the end in sight and the beautiful sweet sound of the bell.

The ding of this particular bell in the world of pediatric cancer signifies the completion of a course of treatment and hopefully a win against a nasty opponent. The ring does not guarantee anything, nor does it erase the trauma and experience of the fight. The bell doesn't eradicate the toxic chemicals that have been pumped through the fighter's body nor does it immune the patient from the potential after-effects of poison killing all the living cells in their body in the hopes of destroying the bad and restarting with new, healthy cells.

I've seen many moms and caregivers post their discontentment of the cancer journey characterized as a battle and our children portrayed as warriors. I, personally, don't have a problem with this analogy. Everyone processes life experiences differently and this analogy may help someone understand what a family is enduring during a cancer diagnosis and treatment.

To further understand what warriors and families endure, I bring you to the basics. Cancer is a fight and a synonym of the word fight is a battle. Merriam-Webster defines battle as "a struggle to succeed or survive". Fighting against cancer is the epitome of struggling to succeed or survive. Round after round of treatment punches the fighter's body in different areas leaving bruises and scars as a reminder that we are fighting poison with poison.

The length of time the bruises take to heal depends on many things out of our control. What others don't necessarily see is the long-term scars that have faded to the point of almost being invisible but still lie at the surface designating the body as a fighter and reminding its wearer that they did indeed struggle to survive the game of life at a point during their existence.

What calling it a fight does not do is explain the absolutely heart-breaking experience of hearing the words "your child has cancer" and having to pick up the pieces of your heart and push them back together in hopes that it can be strong enough to endure the journey, the fight, the battle, (whatever you would like to call it) your child will endure over the next few months, years, or longer. The word "fight" does not fully describe the image of a parent picking up the pieces of their heart and making sure it holds together to be strong for your child. As parents, it's our job to keep our children safe and encourage them along the way. There is no time for your heart to break. God forbid they see the pieces of your heart fall onto the floor.

So, what do you do? You discreetly pick up the pieces and salvage what you can, praying it holds together long enough to support your child and show them how to be brave and strong when it's the only option. I've had to hold my heart together with one hand while holding my child's hand with the other. I've had to watch him endure painful test after painful test, awful side effects, near death experiences, and heartbreak while holding my own heart and praying the patches hold well enough 'til I can fall apart in solitude.

This chapter is not going to be about the hard parts of the journey, however. I have plenty of pages ahead to describe our harrowing journey and the reason I am so vocal in my advocacy for pediatric cancer patients, their parents, and caregivers. The words on the next few pages are going to describe the feeling of the end of treatment.

Notice that I did not say "focus on the happiness of the end of the journey" because there is never happiness without hopelessness and sadness far behind and there is no end of the journey without the threat of after effects or finding out another family is battling this beast. These words will focus on the ringing of the bell, the end of a round, the end of treatment.

On October 3, 2022, we were given the option of finishing treatment after two and a half years due to the ongoing research in the field regarding the length of the maintenance stage of chemo in girls versus boys and some serious side effects Cole battled last spring. In the past, before certain chemo drugs entered the picture, the length of maintenance treatment in T-cell acute lymphoblastic leukemia was two years for girls and three years for boys. As time went on and more research was conducted, there weren't definitive results stating that three years of maintenance was needed for boys.

The protocol changed with B-cell acute lymphoblastic leukemia (ALL) and moved both boys and girls to two years of maintenance therapy. Since protocols, policies, and rules depend on research and definitive results backing the decisions, the changes to treatment protocols are typically made every five years and the official decision to change the length of maintenance for Cole's type of leukemia (T-ALL) did not yet happen.

Due to the impending change in protocol, coupled with side effects Cole experienced caused by the chemotherapy, we were able to end the maintenance phase and ring the bell on October 19, 2022. Our team and the team at a leading children's cancer research hospital who was already following the two-year protocol for Cole's type of cancer felt the decision was based on enough research to stop the maintenance at two years and four months and move to the next phase, after-treatment, especially since chemo was the reason his appendix ruptured, and continuing to suppress his immune system would make him susceptible to possible additional issues.

Making the decision to end treatment earlier than originally planned is one of the most difficult decisions our family faced. It seems our lives have been filled with these types of decisions lately, and the only thing that helped was the peace and guidance of God. I rested in God, used Him as a guide in our lives, and have relied on the signs of the Lord when submerged in difficult waters, and this situation was no different.

After making the decision, I still wrestled and wondered if we were following the correct path. Waking up that morning, I was feeling many emotions. The most prevalent feelings were excitement and nervousness. I was excited for my whole family to finally enter a new phase of this journey.

I felt like we were playing a game of Candy Crush or maybe Candy Land and I was entering a new world of levels. This land was unknown. We had never visited this area and did not know what to expect. We went from the shock of diagnosis pit, to the depths of treatment valley, into the rolling hills of maintenance, and now the glistening peak of the journey was visible, the end of treatment.

This phase of the hypothetical game of Cancer Land or Cancer Crush is like the bonus level where you collect as many coins or candy pieces that you can, but this doesn't mean all the coins are collected and that I wasn't scared but the anticipation of this long-awaited candy castle was what we have been waiting for during the last 33 months.

It was finally here and honestly, I didn't know what to do with myself. Not only was today the long-awaited end of treatment, but it was also the day my son was having his medical port (a device in his chest used to deliver chemo to his body) removed during surgery. Over the last couple of years, we had been down the surgery road a few times but it's always nerve-racking. The bundle of emotions we were all feeling was so hard to describe.

The way that I can make sense of this journey is comparing it to another journey in my life. Ten years ago, when I was 29, I started running. I was on the brink of turning 30 and honestly, I was having a bit of a crisis. I had a six-year-old and a four-year-old, I was a stay-at-home mom with no career, and a hobby/part-time business that was doing semi well. I needed to channel my energy into something that was just for me. So, I started running.

Five years later, I had the idea that I wanted to run a half marathon which was one of those long-lost Candy Land Castles in the distance. Well, I put my mind to running that race and on October, 15 2017, I reached the

Candy Castle. Actually, it was a chocolate factory in Hershey, Pennsylvania during the Hershey Half Marathon in the sweetest place on Earth as they call it.

I am by no means an athletic person, nor was I a runner to any extent. But, I put my mind to finishing the race and that is exactly what I did. At that point in my life, it was one of the hardest things I have ever done. Keep in mind, I finished my college degree and gave birth to two children by this point. But coupled with my anti-athletic nature and snail pace, a half marathon was a Candy Castle in a far, far away land through dungeons, scary forests, and fire-breathing dragons.

Starting slowly and adding mile by mile, I eventually felt like I was going to make it to the race. I made it to 10 miles on several training runs and had a great running partner, my German Shepherd, Laney. Yes, for all of you late 1990s early 2000s teens, I did name my dog after Laney Boggs who is the main character in an epic movie called *She's All That*. Anyway, armed with the knowledge that I was ready for this journey, we checked into our hotel, went to Hershey Park, did some trick-or-treating in Chocolate Town and picked up my race bib on the eve before the big race.

I was so nervous because this was huge. It was something I had talked myself into thinking that I would never ever be able to accomplish. But, I didn't realize that in the past eight months of training, I had become a runner. I transformed into the one thing I never thought I could become. A huge goal completion was within reach and this race was absolutely possible. Even though, when I look back at the night before the race and how mean and nervous I was and how many times I told my husband I wanted to go home, I had the skills, knowledge and training to compete and complete my goal.

The night before the end of treatment, I felt very similar. I was nervous, moody, and I wanted to throw up. I didn't realize that in the past two and a half years we had become warriors and we were now at the point in our journey where we transitioned into survivors. Looking back, I now know that was the moment I finally realized the hardships during the previous two and a half years had given us the skills, knowledge and training to complete this journey and ring that bell. I continually refer to the journey and the cancer fight as "our" journey and "our" fight because our entire family was with Cole every single step of the race and will always continue to be right next to him as long as we are in this world running alongside him.

End of treatment came with many mixed emotions and strong feelings. I have never felt more proud of Cole than in that very moment. All the pain, loss, heartbreak, side effects, pokes and poisons this human being has endured at the age of 17 are daunting to say the least. He has come face-to-face with every opponent with his quiet strength and determined nature, keeping his head up and continuing to move onto the next phase.

Adequately describing the amount of joy, relief, pride, anger, sadness, and heartbreak I felt at one particular moment in time is impossible. Perhaps describing the pure joy and smile that radiated throughout Cole's entire body at the exact moment he grabbed the rope and swung that bell back and forth making the most glorious sound that echoed throughout the clinic hallway will suffice. The smiles and tears on the faces of his nurses, doctors, and child life specialist warmed all our bodies and made everyone glow with joy.

We have witnessed this bell ringing ceremony a few times, mostly behind the clinic door simply listening to the nurses sing with enthusiasm and pride amongst the loud clanging ring of the brass bell in the hallway. Today was a special day. It was Cole's turn. At several points during the journey, I wasn't sure this day would ever come. I had begun to believe it was an enigma, a unicorn that is often talked about as an amazing experience and one of a kind creature, but so rare that I questioned its existence. Our unicorn was finally here. Cole was about to experience something so amazing and realize a goal almost three years in the making.

There is nothing that can prepare you for such a moment. All of my amazing experiences such as graduating high school and college, getting married, having children, receiving various awards, finishing a half marathon and accomplishing other great feats are amazing in and of themselves. However, the experience of my child finishing cancer treatment and marking the event by ringing the bell needs to be placed in a separate category because no comparison will suffice. All of the experiences I have been through in my life and all of my accomplishments do not compare to the pride I felt when I saw the joy on Cole's face after ringing the bell.

Sometimes, well a lot of the time, it's very difficult for me to process the trauma my entire family has been through these last almost three years. I can't even begin to think about how difficult this entire journey has been for Cole who had to live it firsthand, not simply watch it. Watching someone go through such trauma is its own hell, but living it is a whole different level of hell. It's easier for me to process what we have actually been through by comparing our experiences to "normal", everyday things that occur all the time and are expected, such as playing a game of Candy Land or going for a run, training for a race, and reading a book. By normalizing the extenuating circumstances our family has been through these last three years, it is relatable in my own mind.

I hope and pray that you never have to go through a cancer journey yourself or with a family member, but if you did or if you do, I am here. You don't, and will not have to do this alone because Cole and my entire family have been there and will be there for you through our story. I will never stop fighting for others and advocating for all cancer patients, especially children. The fire this journey has ignited in my soul will never go out. I will always fight for all pediatric cancer patients to have the chance to ring the bell. Like I said in the beginning of this chapter, ringing the bell does not erase the trauma. It takes the trauma and sets it on fire, a flame that burns and fuels a fight that resides in the depths of my soul and all the souls of the parents and cancer patients everywhere.

I want nothing more than to make the unicorn of successfully completing treatment a reality for more pediatric cancer patients and their families.

But, how? How can we accomplish such an extraordinary feat? I do not hold all the answers, but I do hold an unending passion and fire for the cause, an ability to advocate and fight for our children, and the knowledge and will to succeed. I hope by sharing our story and combining both my perspective as a parent and Cole's perspective as a teenage cancer survivor we can inspire others to join us in battle, holding that gold flag high as an army against pediatric cancer.

Cole

Ding, Ding, Ding! The sound that signaled my fight against leukemia was won rang out in the hallway of the clinic. The ding of the bell was also the sound that would change my life in more ways than one. The bell ringing was a formal ceremony indicating a new part of my life would begin in a short amount of time. It was a final punch in the battle I had been fighting for almost three years.

More than just a bell, this object signified an end to chemotherapy and hardly as many pokes and prods that I endured previously. Finally, after almost three long years, I was finished with my fight.

The day it really clicked in my mind that treatment was finally over and I could begin to have a more normal life was the day I got my port taken out. This port was actually my second one since the first one was bad and ended up getting infected, meaning I needed to have it taken out, wait six weeks, and have another port put into the same side of my chest.

This port saved my veins and my life but now it was time to have it removed because I would not be needing it anymore. The day it was removed was also the day I would have my last official checkup of active treatment. The end of my battle was sooner than expected due to a pretty bad complication a couple of months before this day. Even though I took my last chemo pill on October 3, 2022, I didn't ring the bell making it real until October 19, 2022.

All of my doctors and nurses brought gifts and sang songs and it was just a very great day. I heard them singing to other kids before me who finished their battle and rang the bell. Finally, it was my turn. They constructed a makeshift banner with my favorite football team, The Seattle Seahawk's stadium as a background. They added pictures of the things I love and they all signed it and wrote notes. I ended up putting this sign up in my room and it still hangs over my TV, months later.

In addition to the banner, I received gift cards, a new basketball, and baked goods from my nurses, doctors and an amazing child life specialist named Rose. These gestures showed they cared. They were all amazing and I was very grateful for all the attention they gave me throughout my fight, but the cause of the celebration was the best part of the day.

I was finally finished with treatment and able to ring the bell. I wasn't nervous to get my port removed, I was actually extremely excited to get it removed and everything went perfectly fine. I got to see some of the same people who removed my last port and one of my favorite nurses was now a nurse in pediatric sedation. He was there for my port removal which made me really happy.

Having the port removed reduced a ton of anxiety. Even though I was grateful for the job the port did of saving my veins and giving me chemo, it also caused stress because I had to be really careful of infections. If I got sick, an infection could go straight to my heart because of the port. So, I had to be extra careful around germs. Having the port removed, in addition to ending the chemo, made me more comfortable and not as anxious. Having the port removal surgery after the bell ringing ceremony was a huge step closer to a normal life.

I barely even noticed that I had been cut open at all. There was only a little slit covered in glue and surgical tape. I decided to keep my port as I weirdly thought it was very cool. One of my favorite teachers told me that she kept her port after her cancer battle, so it was my goal the entire time to keep the port when I finished treatment. I have it in a little jar in my desk next to my gold boxing gloves as a reminder of the fight I endured.

I want to bring you back to the subject of this chapter and the moment I went from fighter to survivor; the act of ringing the bell. Every single time I went into the clinic and got my height, weight, and blood pressure taken, I walked by that bell. The day had finally come when I was able to ring it, and it was the best sound I've ever heard.

In the past almost three years, I seemingly had forgotten how to live a normal life. I became used to staying extremely safe because a germ harmless to most could make me very sick. Everyone was pretty careful with COVID, so during the pandemic I didn't feel so different from others, but that was now mostly over and I still had treatment, so while people were getting back to normal, I wasn't yet ready until now.

In addition to germs, I also had to be careful of bruises that could lead my parents to believe I had low platelets and would need a platelet transfusion. I wasn't allowed to eat any fresh vegetables or any raw foods. Everything had to be cooked very well, including my steak, which was definitely not the tastiest way to cook steak. I would not be able to eat anything that wasn't overcooked and overheated. All steps were taken to make sure I didn't get sick because we did not want to end up staying in the hospital any more than we already had or deal with potential life-threatening complications like an infection.

Weeks after I rang the bell and officially stopped treatment, I still followed those same rules. I was still very paranoid of getting sick and made sure to stay extra careful. It took a while until I was able to fully adjust to a semi normal life, back to being how it had been before my diagnosis.

At first, it was very weird for my life to be back to normal. It wasn't completely back to normal, however. I still needed to go to the hospital once a month for checkups and would also need to keep getting blood work, but it was much more normal than it had been for the past couple of years. I began to start getting out as much as I could again, trying to adapt to the norms of society even though the last couple years of my life had been anything but normal.

The ring of the bell allowed me to hang out with my friends more and go to more places than when I was under treatment. It felt awesome because it was like I had been in a little bubble the last almost three years, afraid of getting sick due to my weak immune system. The ding that bell made allowed me to break out of that bubble and signified the start of a new beginning. Even though I had more freedom, I realized not everything was back to normal.

I still felt pretty weak. It took a little while until my energy was back to how it used to be but every month I began to feel more and more like my old self. My blood counts and immune system would take time to recover so I would still need to be careful for a couple of months and make sure I stayed as sanitary as possible to avoid unnecessary sickness which would set back my immune system recovery time. As I'm writing this, my counts have still not fully recovered but are definitely way better than they were during treatment, maintenance, and even a couple of months ago.

I feel more energized and I'm now able to fully participate in any sport I would like to play. Having most of my energy back feels great. I'm now able to play the sports I loved again, at full speed and I'm looking forward to my senior football season this fall.

I think most kids undergoing treatment feel so defeated because they can't participate in the sports or activities they loved before they were diagnosed. It was really hard for me to watch my friends play football and go sit in the audience at ice hockey games while others were on the ice having fun. I missed three years of sports, but I'm excited to be able to play again.

It's important for kids battling cancer to remember that at some point your energy will come back and your drive to do the things you love will also come back. It's all about completing the fight at hand so that when it's over you can enjoy yourself again, have fun, and do the things you love to do most in this world. Whether you love sports like I do, or you love to make music or draw remember that even if you can't focus on these activities while in your fight, they will still be waiting when you're ready.

After my treatment ended, I became more involved with sports and all I want to do is learn more and study the sports I love to watch and play. I believe this happens to others as well when they can finally put effort into something besides fighting the cancer. This is a very good thing because you no longer have to focus your energy towards beating this awful disease and can focus that energy toward things you love to do. This is a blessing after the fight.

I'm currently a couple of months post my end of treatment celebration and my life has continued to improve drastically. All of the treatments, hospital visits, tests, and admissions became a norm in my life and it made me very angry because I had no control over my own life. It was a constant cycle of getting treatment, getting sick from the side effects, and repeating the cycle. Now that time has passed, I see how it was worth it to push through all the treatments and hard times and get over the mountain to the other side. Although once you climb the mountain everything on the other side may not be exactly as you remember before diagnosis life, it is better and it does get better after treatment.

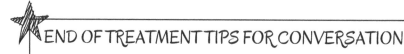

Parents/Caregivers

End of Treatment is its own separate journey and new territory for everyone. Give grace and follow their lead. If a huge party is not what they need, acknowledge it and support them (I focused on the bell ringing and celebrating with family, friends and supporters because that is what Cole chose to do, but each person is different and will choose a different way to commemorate such a momentous accomplishment).

Have a conversation asking how they want to celebrate this milestone. Our children lose control over many things in treatment. This should be a decision for them and supported by us.

Supporters

Instead of saying "you must be so happy he is finally cancer free" to a parent of a pediatric cancer warrior, say: "I know you must be having a lot of emotions during this new phase in your journey. I am very happy to hear he/she has reached this milestone. If you ever need anything, don't hesitate to reach out. I might not understand what you are going through but I can listen".

It's important to realize that remission or cancer free aren't cure-all words. They don't erase the anxiety, trauma, and side effects. The journey is ongoing, even after the bell rings. So, even though ringing the bell is a momentous victory, nothing is black and white in the pediatric or adult cancer worlds. Acknowledging that joy and excitement aren't the only emotions families are feeling during this stage is important.

CHAPTER 2

Blindsided by a Life-Changing Diagnosis

You are never prepared to hear the word *cancer* when it comes to your health or a family member's health.

Laura

I know because I heard this word three times in two years with three different family members. Each time, I was completely taken off-guard in a traumatic and chaotic way. My mind never went to a possible cancer diagnosis in each of these instances for very different reasons.

When Cole was diagnosed, I didn't let my mind entertain cancer as a possibility. When my dad was diagnosed, I didn't want to think it could be cancer because we were already in the fight with Cole and it couldn't possibly be happening to our family again. The third time, with my stepdad, everything progressed so quickly I didn't have time to think of anything, let alone help yet a third family member through a cancer battle. For these pages, I am focusing on our first cancer journey, Cole's diagnosis and treatment.

I previously discussed the end of treatment, ringing the bell, and all the emotions that go along with reaching this point in a cancer journey. I chose to start the very first chapter of our story with this topic for a reason. An explanation for why I would start at the end is summarized in one simple but powerful word: *hope*. I want to give families who are in the deep and dark parts of the journey a bit of light in the darkness. I have seen different outcomes in each of my family members' stories, but I have always experienced beauty in the darkness and glimpses of light in even the most remote caverns of despair. I wanted to show you our light and lend it to you as you continue reading our story. I am hopeful that when reaching the heartache and turmoil we experienced you remember the light in the beginning and keep going, one page at a time.

Sharing the hard parts is necessary and equal to, if not more important, than the triumph because I've noticed that trauma and heartbreak move people to do something and act upon their emotions by helping others and giving them the hope that they, too, will experience light in the darkness. It's important to realize the bell does not erase the experience. It is another experience in and of itself.

By describing how it felt to be finished with treatment first, I aim to prepare you for the journey which is often hard to watch, listen to, or read. My hope is that as you walk beside us during this journey, you remember where Cole and I are today. We are in a stable place right now even though there are a whole set of different challenges in our after-treatment world. We are so grateful for every moment of togetherness our family is able to experience in this life.

As a result of our experience, we developed a fire and passion for helping others. I always say, "If I can make this journey even a little bit easier for anyone going through it, I am honored to do so". I don't want the journey to be in vain or wasted. All the knowledge and experience we've gained through the heartache and despair cannot sit idle.

Cancer, especially your child's cancer, is one of those experiences, in my opinion, that you could and would change if given the chance. I'm sure you've heard the expression "even though it was difficult, if I could go back in time, I wouldn't change anything". Well, in this case, I am grateful for the experience and ability to help others, but I would absolutely change and take it away if given the chance. This is one journey that I hope you never personally take, and I would hang up my boots and erase all the pain and suffering my family has endured in the last three years if I were given the proverbial magic wand.

All wishes and wands aside, I realize it's not possible. Magic, genies, and wands only exist in fairy tales and our imagination. Our reality won't change, but I feel a great responsibility to try and change the future journey of a family by using our words and experiences to aid in better research, more funding, new less toxic medication, less side effects, less mental and physical trauma and an overall easier terrain than we endured. I am going to attempt to describe how it felt prior to, during, and immediately after the first few days after diagnosis. There are no words to describe the intensity of my emotions, but if reliving this experience will help others, it is worth it. Here we go…

In the fall of 2019, my previously healthy 14-year-old son had an amazing 8th grade football season filled with pick sixes and epic jukes and tackles. I picked up my football lingo through exposure and Google. For those of you who are not football term literate, this equates to all the amazing things you see a player do on television resulting in the crowd cheering with amazement of the player's skills and dedication.

I try really hard to watch football and sound like I know what is going on, but I also realize that I am fooling no one. I was a field hockey player for a couple of years in junior high, so when the boys were playing ice hockey, I understood that a heck of a lot more and actually felt like I knew what was happening and wasn't standing around watching something completely foreign and unfamiliar.

My husband, however, was a gifted football player for a locally famous high school with an equally famous head coach so he clearly speaks fluent football terms on a daily basis and even coached Cole for one year during midget football. Parents who coach their children, you are amazing individuals.

Anyway, Cole has always loved tackling people. Even when he was a toddler, I remember him jamming out to The Foo Fighters, *The Pretender*, and running as fast as he could into our ancient floor model big screen TV circa 2008. Dave Grohl, you were tackled on a daily basis as you belted out the lyrics to his favorite song. There is even a long-lost camcorder video out there somewhere proving my story and if I ever find it, it's going to be played at Cole's graduation, wedding, and shown to everyone we know.

Football and sports in general have always been a passion for Cole, so when he complained of leg pain, vision changes, and showed excessive bruising during the season, we thought he was putting his all into practice, during games, and simply overworked playing both offensive and defensive positions during the season. Another possible explanation for the leg pain was a Lyme disease diagnosis the previous summer. So, no deafening alarm bells were ringing with any of these symptoms.

Upon the end of the season, the symptoms intensified, and by Christmas, Cole developed some alarming lumps under his arms. At this point, he was still working out by lifting and running five miles on the treadmill daily. So, when he was taken to the acute care center on January 12, 2020, I wasn't extremely concerned. To be honest, I was relieved when he was diagnosed with an inflamed sweat gland and put on antibiotics. I should also mention that he often had small bumps and inflamed sweat glands throughout the season, but they were starting to get more severe.

The next day, the headaches started. Upon a Google search of the antibiotic he was taking, the internet listed headache near the top of the side effect list. So that was the culprit, right? This is what we thought, but on the second day of the headaches, we called his pediatrician. Something wasn't right. At this point, lymph nodes were popping out on his neck, he was very tired, and the headaches were extremely bad.

When we entered the pediatrician's office and saw his baby and childhood doctor, I was comforted in the statement that she fully believed this was mono because it was presenting like the virus, and they were seeing many cases during this particular time. She was going to run a full blood panel in addition to the mono test just in case because sometimes it could be more, and she wanted to be safe. The doctor reassured us once again as we were leaving the exam room that she thought it was mono, but she was crossing all T's and dotting I's by doing a full blood panel.

Reliving and rewriting the experience of that day brings back such strong emotions watching my son in so much pain. It's like I am watching myself through a window or on a television screen sitting next to Cole in the waiting room of the hospital, waiting for him to be called to the lab for blood work. He was holding his head and unable to stay awake in the waiting room. We sat there, in that room, and waited for his name to pop up on the screen with the accompanying ding that a registration desk was free and ready to process his lab order.

We finally heard the ding and saw his name flash on the screen, walked to registration, and minutes later a phlebotomist came to get us for the lab work. Before this day, Cole never had blood taken and was a little nervous, but did well.

Upon arriving home, he didn't even make it to his bedroom. He walked to the couch and immediately fell asleep. At one point, he woke and began to vomit blood. Nothing like this had ever happened to my children, myself, or anyone in my family so I immediately called the doctor who reassured me that it wasn't concerning unless it was a large amount, and it could be a result of what she still believed was the mono virus. The bloodwork wasn't back yet, but she would call when it finished processing.

I remember thinking in the back of my mind that this was not mono. The doctor was incorrect and I wasn't sure what it was, but I wasn't convinced that the illness plaguing my son and rendering him completely exhausted and borderline incapacitated could be a virus, the so-called "kissing disease". However, I never in my worst nightmares believed cancer was the evil plaguing my son.

Not even an hour after I called the doctor with my concerns that my son was vomiting blood and still very sick, I received the absolutely worst phone call of my life. Cole was still lying on the couch asleep when the phone rang. I walked into the bedroom with my husband close behind because we knew it was a call that the blood test was back and we would finally know what we were dealing with at this point.

The Dr. asked if I was somewhere I could sit down. I don't even remember if I was thinking at that point because all I remember doing is sitting on the edge of my bed immediately and my husband following suit with his ear on my shoulder, close to the phone so he could hear the sharp daggers of the words our beloved pediatrician was about to throw into my heart.

I do not remember the exact words she uttered, but I do remember something to the effect of "the blood results came back indicating leukemia" and I was to take Cole to the ER immediately where a pediatric oncologist would be waiting. It wasn't necessary to take an ambulance, but I needed to leave right away and get him there immediately. I started shaking and crying while my husband held my crumpling body still.

Now I know why people recommend that you sit down before giving you shocking news. If we had not been sitting, I would have fallen immediately. Since I was sitting, I didn't have the urge to throw myself onto the floor and crumple into the fetal position trying to hold my body together. I simply slumped into my husband and inquired about the next steps.

I immediately walked outside in the blustery cold upon hanging up the phone. As I look back, I didn't even feel the cold, January, Pennsylvania temperature on my coatless torso. I felt nothing but immense panic and a tightness in my chest as my heart was breaking into a million pieces.

I reached out to the first person who entered my mind and who I always reach to for comfort during a trying time. Since I am an only child, I have no biological siblings, but I grew up very close to my cousins Jessie and Aaron. Our moms are sisters, so we have the same maternal grandparents and grew up together, sharing many milestones and life experiences along the way. Jess is closer in age to me, she's Cole's godmother, and we think of each other as sisters. She is the person I turn to for advice and comfort and this time was no different.

I remember asking her if she was busy and then immediately cried and yelled that they thought Cole had leukemia with complete disregard of the fact that she was, in fact, busy and currently at the salon with her head in a shampoo bowl finally pampering herself after a long day working at the hospital. Jess works in the operating room at the hospital where Cole was treated, which proved a blessing in many ways throughout treatment.

Also, I found out later that evening her stylist, who was within listening distance of this entire conversation, just learned her husband had leukemia and he recently started treatments to prepare for a bone marrow transplant.

Upon hearing my panic, she immediately urged Jess out of the chair and told her to pay later so she could be there for us as we entered this unknown territory, a road she was unfortunately traveling with her family as well. The grace her stylist showed was the first of many acts of complete kindness, empathy, and compassion we witnessed through the last few years.

Knowing that my cousin was going to meet us at the hospital, I woke Cole, got him dressed, and escorted him to my truck where we drove the eight miles to the hospital in the dark as I contemplated what was going to happen in the next few hours. My husband stayed with our younger son, Kaden, who was 11 at the time, waiting for my parents to take him to their house since we did not know how long we would be gone and anticipated not returning to our home for several days.

It was dark and around 7 PM when we were driving down our country road. It was a straight line to the hospital with only one turn in the entire journey. I mentioned before that we live in Pennsylvania and if you know anything about this state and the country roads in rural areas, you know that deer tend to be along these roads. It seems like there was a cluster of deer every mile I drove who picked up their heads and stared into my truck, letting me know they were guarding the road and we would safely get to our destination even though I couldn't keep my head straight at this point.

I fully believe this was my Pap. We had an incredibly close bond since I was the first grandchild and my grandparents watched me while my mom worked and I wasn't in school. He passed away in 2012 and I often see birds, turkeys, and deer that just seem to know me really well when I'm going through a hard spot in life. He was an avid hunter and outdoors man so the fact that he would use wildlife to let me know he was watching over my family just makes sense. It may seem crazy, but there was just a feeling that I got on that drive that someone was watching over and protecting us at that particular moment in time.

When we arrived at the hospital, I parked in the lot and was greeted by a sullen Jess. She and I both held it together for Cole, but I immediately saw the fear in her eyes. As I look back, I know I was still in complete shock and unable to process what was happening and believe that was the reason we were both able to be completely emotionless as we walked to the Emergency Room on that dark, cold, January night.

I also can't believe that a couple of hours after walking into the ER, we learned the results of Cole's bloodwork which were completely shocking and explain why the doctor said we needed to get there immediately. His potassium level was a nine. To put this number into context, grown adults can have heart attacks at a lower level.

The amount of leukemia blasts (leukemia cells that were rapidly dividing and multiplying) in his blood along with the elevated white blood cell count contributed to the rise in potassium which would ultimately land us in the PICU (Pediatric Intensive Care Unit) for five days.

This strong and courageous teen walked, unassisted, into the ER with a white blood cell count of 326,000, a potassium of nine, and low platelets signified by a petechiae rash covering his legs. The petechiae looks like little red specks all over the skin and it was shocking to notice as Cole laid on the ER stretcher.

I know I just threw out a ton of medical terms which roll off my tongue with ease at this point in our journey, so I want to explain a little more.

A normal white blood cell count in a healthy person is 8,000-10,000 while my sons was 326,000. Also, the normal range for potassium is 3.4-4.7 for a healthy person under the age of 18. Cole's was nine, and even though it was a little more than double the norm, a level of nine is extremely dangerous to the heart. Cole's platelets were also 11. To put this into perspective, platelets under 50 qualify you for a platelet transfusion at our treating hospital and low platelets cause all sorts of havoc like nose bleeds, petechiae (the red rash on his legs), easy bruising and bleeding.

The numbers indicated in his results told the story of how sick Cole had become in the last week. We had no idea. Five days before the ER walk, Cole was running five miles per day and lifting to stay in shape after finishing football. Now, he was fighting for his life. Three days before the ER walk, infected sweat glands were thought to be the culprit only to find out that it wasn't infected sweat glands at all. The inflamed sweat glands were later diagnosed as hidradenitis suppurativa, an autoimmune skin condition which is annoying and notoriously difficult to treat. These disgusting pimple-like bumps were a separate diagnosis which initially alerted us that something wasn't right in his body.

Prior to January 15, 2020, the thought was that Cole had mono or a similar virus that was making him sick. Prior to the phone call from our pediatrician, the silent eight-mile drive to the hospital, and the walk to the ER, our lives were normal, and our stress was normal. I clearly remember that day as the day our lives changed forever and the level of stress, anxiety, and fear in our lives was about to enter a new realm. This day created a clear line of before and after cancer in our lives.

The walk into the emergency room signified the beginning of a battle we were unprepared to face. Cole, Jess and I walked in together, talking like it was just another day. At that moment, I didn't know how sick Cole truly was, but I was about to find out. The numbers I discussed previously signified that the leukemia was allowed to grow and divide like crazy, either due to time or aggressiveness (we can't be sure).

We were processed through the emergency department quickly and informed that Cole was going to be admitted to Children's Three which we would later find out is the pediatric oncology floor. At some point during the night, I realized I couldn't keep it together any longer and knowing me so well, Jess could tell and took me into her break room and gave me a cup of water. By the time I finished drinking, a text rang through on my phone signaling us that Cole's room was ready.

At this point, we got Cole settled in his room and met the oncologist to have a discussion. With every ounce of my being, I held out hope that the blood test was wrong, the results were mixed up and the leukemia diagnosis was a mistake.

My mom, Jess, Josh, and I walked down the hallway with the oncologist who would later save Cole's life and his resident, a lovely individual who has been a doctor for a short two years, but had the grace of a veteran physician. We entered "The Quiet Room" down the hallway. It was a small room with a beautiful blue and teal stained glass window on one wall to create privacy. I remember sitting along the outside wall, my back to the window next to my husband, and holding on to his hand for dear life, support and anything else that would give me the strength to get through this super difficult and life-altering conversation.

Our doctor and his resident were at the other end of the room almost like we were all seated at a table and they occupied the head of the table. My husband and I were on one side of the table with my cousin Jess and my mom on the other. Even though the oncologist was just about as far as he could get from me, his words shot directly to my heart, creating hole after hole with their vileness. I can't remember any of these words, but I do remember he was explaining everything, giving his medical opinion about what was going on, and talking about the next steps.

I was so overwhelmed with the information, I asked him to stop because I needed a moment. Speaking up for myself was extremely uncharacteristic and not at all something I normally do in this type of situation, but I was experiencing such a wave of nausea I needed his words to stop and get some air into my lungs.

I felt extremely sweaty. The air was a thousand pounds, and my throat had the lump you get before vomiting. I looked around the room for a trash can but there was none in site. The only thoughts in my head were that I was going to embarrass myself and my family by puking in front of everyone. Do I run? Where do I go? I needed to calm down and stop this before I actually threw up.

Thankfully, I was able to breathe and realized I was probably holding my breath the entire time our doctor was giving us the diagnosis and discussing next steps. After getting a few cleansing breaths in my lungs and swallowing the lump in my throat I was ready to hear the rest like a carsick toddler who needed the doctor to pull over on the side of the road until I could catch my bearings and continue the drive.

Embarrassment was an understatement. I never experienced anything like what happened in that room before or since, but I also never experienced someone telling me my son had cancer. The whole time before the doctor's words hit my soul, I still had hope that this was a dream or a terrible mistake.

My mind went back in time to when my cousin Jess (who was present in the room) was two years old and she was very sick and her parents heard the same words we just heard "Your child has leukemia". They diagnosed her.

Keep in mind, this was the early 1990s and leukemia was pretty much a death sentence. I cannot imagine what her parents were going through. Jess was their first and only child at this point and very sick. Not only did they hear those words like I did, but the options to treat their child, at that point were not ideal or very successful.

It turned out that in Jess's case, it was a mistake. The doctors made a mistake in the diagnosis. The illness that plagued my cousin as a toddler was NOT leukemia. In a weird twist of events, it turns out my cousin had mono and a sinus infection at the same time.

Now, if you remember, mono is what Cole's pediatrician originally thought was plaguing my son, so it was totally possible they were mistaken, right? It could still be mono. Doctors have made this mistake before because our family experienced it in the past.

Due to the history with Jess, my family kept reminding me it could be a mistake. Hearing the doctor's words and now knowing there was no mistake brought me to my knees. We weren't the lucky ones this time. Those words made it so real and hit me in the depths of my soul. Cole, in fact, did have leukemia. The words the doctor threw at that beautiful stained glass window were correct and I imagined it shattering in a million pieces all over the hallway just like my heart.

How was I going to tell my sweet boy that he had leukemia? What could I possibly say to give him the courage and strength for the fight he was about to endure? I really didn't know what to do, nor do I remember exactly what I said, but I do remember Cole's reaction of quiet strength and determination and the fact that this child did not shed one tear or yell one word of anger.

After returning to Cole's room from the "quiet room" that screamed daggers, things are fuzzy. I do remember KJ, the sweet third shift nurse with over 40 years of experience and compassion in her heart for every one of her patients. As KJ was getting Cole comfortable and giving him the medication ordered by his doctors, we were told his oncologist and the PICU doctors felt he needed to stay there due to his potassium level.

There was no time to get comfortable. I don't think we were in Children's Three for an hour before we were being moved to the intensive care unit. Since the cancer is acute lymphoblastic leukemia, the acute part signifies a rapid onset. Cole's cancer cells were dividing extremely fast and causing all kinds of havoc in his body, including the high potassium which was extremely dangerous and could cause an immediate heart attack for anyone, regardless of age or overall health. The PICU allowed 24/7 care and observation.

When I heard the name PICU, I remembered a classmate in my Masters of School Counseling program from which I graduated one month prior to Cole's diagnosis, was a third shift nursing assistant in the PICU. What were the chances that she would be working tonight? One in a million or even less since she was part-time, but the thought still crossed my mind.

The nurses detached Cole from his monitors and IV pole and got him ready for transport. With my husband and me next to the hospital bed, he was transported to the PICU two floors down. As soon as the automatic door opened, there was my classmate. Immediately upon seeing her face, she came running to me and I to her. We were hugging and I was crying and spewing out all of the details from the last few hours. If you are keeping track, this is the third sign from God in just one evening, letting me know that I wasn't alone and He was there to guide me by sending familiar faces and comfort.

The first night in the PICU, we didn't sleep much at all, maybe an hour, while Cole was getting CT scans and echocardiograms. The tests were being done to see if the leukemia was causing other issues in his body. I distinctly remember drifting off on the hard, pullout lounge chair with the sandpaper sheets and waking suddenly with the feeling that someone was sitting on my chest and I couldn't breathe. I shot up to a sitting position immediately and began to gasp for breath. I was covered in sweat and struggling to breathe the sterile, dry, hospital air. The "elephant on my chest" experience was frightening, and only the first time of several similar episodes during those harrowing days in the hospital.

When Cole was diagnosed in January 2020, it was prior to COVID, temperature checks, screening at the front door, and masks required throughout the hospital. Since our diagnosis was pre-COVID, we were able to have visitors. I cannot express how much it helped us get through diagnosis and our first admission.

Having our family and Cole's friends visit gave us the strength and support we so desperately needed. One of those visitors was another angel sent to me in my time of need. I met her a few months prior to Cole's diagnosis when she was hired at the school where I was completing my internship hours to become a school counselor. It just so happened that prior to accepting a position at the school district, she was a grief counselor in the children's hospital where Cole was currently admitted and later treated. She worked closely with oncology patients and families for over 14 years. Upon hearing about Cole's diagnosis, Mary came directly to the PICU, embracing me and pulling me into a quiet room where she comforted me, explained the next steps, and introduced me to everyone I would need to know in our area of the hospital.

I can compare pre-COVID and post-COVID admissions and could not imagine initial diagnosis occurring after COVID protocols were put in place. The visitors, cards, gift baskets, and daily check-ins and coffee from my cousin is what encouraged us all and not only helped Cole, my husband and me during our stay, but our younger son Kaden and immediate family who were extremely concerned and shocked, were able to see Cole which helped ease their minds as well.

Our subsequent admissions were very different, especially immediately after COVID protocols in March of 2020. Complete isolation, COVID testing due to a fever upon admission, and no contact with anyone for more than a couple of minutes were awful. I couldn't leave the room, both Cole and I had to wear masks in the room at all times, and didn't interact with anyone other than each other.

I talk often about support and how we couldn't have gotten through the last three plus years without our friends and family behind us every step of the way. I have mixed feelings regarding the help we were offered. I believe this is due to the fact our family is very private and keeps things to ourselves. So, suddenly having everything that was occurring in our family made public was a little unnerving to say the least.

Everyone reacts differently when faced with a childhood cancer diagnosis or hearing of someone close facing this monster. There is no roadmap or etiquette guide to cancer. It's messy, evil, unpredictable, and downright nasty. The tips at the end of each chapter aim to show some helpful advice and tricks, but it's not an all-inclusive list. Give yourself grace, act how you are drawn to act and if you need a break just to be with your family, take one.

I couldn't even post about Cole's diagnosis for weeks. I wasn't sure I was going to let everyone know what was going on in our lives but at the moment, I decided to share our story, I knew we needed the cheerleaders and supporters behind us. Cole needed to know he was loved, cared for, and not alone in his journey.

So, I pushed aside my pride and sought out support. Our church, friends, family, teachers, coworkers, and the community rallied behind us and helped us through the first hospital stay and many other hardships we endured during the process.

Describing step-by-step the events that occurred on diagnosis day almost three years to the date afterwards, is surreal. Looking back on that very first day, I had no clue what we would face throughout our cancer journey. I can say with utmost certainty that the one thing that got us through our journey besides prayers, is support. The kindness, compassion, and well-wishes from others gave us fuel for the fight. The hospital staff and the relationships we have built with the nurses, staff, child life specialists, and doctors are without a doubt, what comforted us the most.

From that very first day when I ran into a friend in the PICU, the next day having another friend drop everything and comfort me, and running into two long-time friends in the atrium café who happened to work at the large hospital, to the days that followed with amazing nurses that distracted Cole from everything and kept him as comfortable as possible, our support squad helped us through the dark, trauma, and uncertainty while giving us the support, excellent care, and guidance needed to move forward.

Cole

The days before diagnosis were filled with hardships. I had a terrible headache that made it almost unbearable to do anything. I also felt extremely tired and I just really did not feel like myself. A week or so before I was diagnosed, lymph nodes around my neck had also become enlarged, but as a kid I didn't think too much about it since I had no idea what could cause something like this to happen.

At that point I also felt pretty much normal. I felt a little bit sick, like I had a cold or the flu, and just didn't feel completely fine. Days before my diagnosis, this started to change. At this point, I could barely eat any food. I didn't eat lunch at school. The most I could eat was a granola bar. All of a sudden, one day, a switch flipped and I began to feel very sick. Things changed extremely quickly.

Up to this point, I was very active, working out and running every day. I had also just finished my 8th grade football season and was probably in the best shape I had ever been in. However, as the days passed, I couldn't really eat anything or even move, let alone run and workout. I just spent most of my time sleeping.

The day I ended up hospitalized for the first time and later diagnosed with T-cell acute lymphoblastic leukemia started off just as any other day. I woke up and got on the bus to head to school and went about my day like normal. I did have a headache, but thought it would hopefully go away. The headache did not let up. It persisted throughout the day and instead of getting better, it got progressively worse. The pain got to the point where I could no longer focus on schoolwork, and I could barely stay awake.

At the beginning of the second to the last period of the day, I went to the nurse and was sent back to class after receiving medicine for my headache. I would eventually learn that this was not a regular headache, it was a migraine caused by the leukemia in my body, and the medicine I was given did nothing to help ease the pain. Halfway through this period I could not stand to be in class anymore. I couldn't focus, I was in pain, and extremely uncomfortable.

I had to get out of class and asked to go to the bathroom. I would end up staying in the bathroom for the remainder of the period. I was just trying to wait it out. The final period of the day had finally arrived and again, I spent the entire period waiting in the bathroom. After the school day ended, I gathered my things and headed to my bus. Unfortunately, my bus ride was not a short one, I was one of the last kids to get off the bus. I spent almost of the entire bus ride sleeping and trying to deal with the unbearable headache.

Once I arrived home, my mom took me straight to the doctor. I remember being in so much pain and being so tired. The doctor said she thought I had mono which can make you very tired. So, I thought that's what was making me so sick. I had to go get my blood taken to see if it really was mono. So, after the appointment we went downstairs and waited to get the blood drawn. I never had blood taken before, so I was a little nervous that it was going to hurt. Now, I am so used to it, because I have been poked so many times since then it doesn't bother me too much anymore.

I don't even remember getting home and lying down, but I know I was so tired that I couldn't keep my eyes open. I fell asleep on the couch and started to feel really nauseous and went to throw up. When I threw up in the bathroom, I was throwing up blood which was scary.

I also remember my mom being really worried and trying to figure out what was going on. Everything is pretty fuzzy the night of diagnosis because I was so exhausted and my head was pounding even after taking medicine. I do remember my mom waking me up and telling me we needed to go to the hospital. On the drive she told me they thought I had leukemia. We weren't sure what was going on, but the doctors were going to work to make me feel better.

I could tell that my mom was really upset, and it didn't really sink in that when she said "leukemia", she meant cancer. I just remember feeling sick and wanting my head to stop hurting. When I got to the emergency room my godmother Jessie was there. When I saw her, I knew something was wrong because she doesn't work at night. Jessie distracted me and kept talking to me while my mom checked us in. We went right into the emergency room, and I was put on a bed right away. I didn't even have to wait in the waiting room.

I don't remember too much about the emergency department, but I do remember my friend's mom, who was a nurse at the hospital, came into my room and talked to us for a little bit. After the doctor looked at me and they put an IV in my arm, my room upstairs was ready.

I had never stayed in the hospital before, so I didn't really know what to expect. When I realized I was going to be admitted, my first thought was that I might be there for a couple of days until I felt better, then I would be able to go home. However, I didn't realize my leukemia diagnosis would mean I needed to stay almost two weeks and be in treatment for over three years with a few hospital stays in the mix.

My first stay in the hospital wasn't filled with any worry or anxiety because I was still in shock. At this point, I couldn't grasp what was happening and what my diagnosis meant. My regular doctor thought it was mono, so I thought I would be sick a couple of weeks. I never expected it to be leukemia.

I no sooner got to the emergency room and got changed into a gown than I was transported up to a room. When I arrived on Children's Three, the oncology floor, I met my first oncologist Dr. Yohannes. He would be the doctor that saved my life and made the right decisions for the beginning of my treatment. He tried to describe everything so I could understand what was going to happen and he did a great job and answered any questions I had, always keeping me informed of what he was doing.

I really did not know much about leukemia, cancer, or the hospital in general. I had no clue what was going to happen in the first couple of days. I was in so much pain from my headache and things were happening so quickly that I couldn't focus on anything or think about the treatment I would need during the next couple of years.

I was also told I needed a port placed in my chest and would need chemotherapy a few times a week for a while. I never had bloodwork, an IV, or a broken bone, let alone surgery, so I was nervous to have the port placed. My godmother worked in Interventional Radiology, the department that places ports at my hospital, and was able to explain everything to me and introduce me to the doctors and nurses that were going to be doing the surgery.

Not only would I get the port put in my chest, but I would get my first spinal tap with chemo and a bone marrow aspiration which resulted in my first spinal headache. These headaches are unlike anything I ever experienced, even worse than the headaches I had at diagnosis. I couldn't sit up, walk, or even move when the spinal headache started.

Everything that happened when I was diagnosed happened very quickly and I didn't even get the chance to process everything until I was discharged and received chemo in the clinic. I do remember being very upset about losing my hair and I even told my parents I didn't want treatment if my hair was going to fall out. Now, I realize treatment was absolutely necessary, but I was worried about this new journey and didn't know what to expect.

One thing that did help during those first few days in the hospital is visits from my family and friends. My two best friends at the time were very worried about me and wanted to come visit me in the PICU. They put on yellow gowns and wore masks just to spend time with me in those early days of my diagnosis. Since my friend's mom was a nurse in the hospital she explained what they should expect so they weren't nervous. We sat and played video games just like we always did and suddenly things didn't seem so scary.

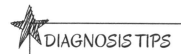

DIAGNOSIS TIPS

Parents/Caregivers

Take it one moment at a time. Slow down and breathe. This is easier said than done, but focus on the here and now. Don't look forward. Don't look back. Sometimes you may need to take it minute by minute and that's ok. Eventually you can get to taking it one day at a time and even further as time progresses.

Let people help, but only allow what makes you comfortable and tell others what you need if you're able.

Ask questions. Ask lots of questions and advocate for your child or the child under your care.

Supporters

Be specific in your support...instead of asking what you can do, ask if you can provide a meal or what their favorite restaurant is. Families are making a ton of really hard decisions and may not be able to think straight to tell someone what they need.

Give the family space. Offer your support, but don't push. Know when to support and when to step back. Take cues from the family as to what they need.

Sometimes a meal or a card left on their doorstop or at the hospital can be monumental to a newly diagnosed family.

Be there. Check in once in a while, to offer support, a meal, a gift card, or to just listen.

CHAPTER 3

Beginnings Come in all Forms

Some are hard, some are easy, some are wished for, and some are feared.

Laura

The beginning of our treatment journey starts the day after diagnosis. Since Cole's white blood count and potassium were extremely high, the doctors knew it was necessary to start treatment immediately to prevent any further kidney damage and begin wiping out the cancer. His kidneys did suffer some damage and the pediatric nephrologist described it like a bad sunburn and they would support his kidneys with fluids and keep an eye on things to make sure the damage didn't get worse.

This was the first encouraging news we heard because there was talk amongst the doctors about using dialysis to support Cole's kidneys and rid his system of toxins. Thankfully it wasn't needed because his treatment team monitored his potassium, placed him on a special diet, and administered fluids around the clock.

The special diet stunk. There wasn't too much Cole was allowed to have and we were surprised to find out potassium is in so many more things than bananas. Coupled with the steroids, mealtime was less than pleasant and we were counting down the time until more food options were on the menu.

Fluids were another story altogether. Cole's legs and feet blew up like a water balloon ready to burst. His feet were so filled to the brim with the extra fluid that he even required the largest pair of non-slip socks the hospital carried. I still have those enormous, bright, yellow, pieces of fabric that made his feet look like huge bananas hanging off the ends of his swollen tree trunk legs.

Since we were admitted in the evening, preparations to begin treatment didn't start until the next day. After the middle of the night echo and CT scan to make sure the leukemia didn't impact his brain (thank God it did not), Cole visited a department in the hospital called Interventional Radiology in the morning to have a power port placed in his chest to attempt to preserve his veins and shield them from the burning chemo. Immediately after placement, the port was put to work, delivering the first dose of chemotherapy. Cole also received a dose of chemo directly to his spinal fluid and a bone marrow aspiration to determine how many leukemic cells were in his body and the exact type of his leukemia to further narrow his treatment plan.

Everything progressed extremely fast which didn't allow us time to come out of the shock and really process what was going to happen. I am extremely grateful for the route our journey took. I realize that many families were not in this situation and treatment did not begin immediately. Having time to digest what was about to happen and the trauma we just experienced would have created more anguish and anxiety. A wait between diagnosis and treatment would raise the level of anxiety to unbearable in our specific circumstance.

Since we were already in crisis mode, with our stress response heightened, we were able to progress through those first few days in the hospital in a trauma induced haze. I am eternally grateful for the fast diagnosis and treatment.

One of Cole's doctors who has been in the field almost 30 years, described the stages families and patients go through upon diagnosis. This angel of a doctor described the look of newly diagnosed families resembling deer illuminated and frozen in the glow of a vehicle's headlights which often occurs when the animal comes face to face with a moving vehicle. The doctor realized it's necessary to give the families grace and repeat many of the instructions given those first weeks because the shock is easy to see from an outsider's perspective. The tell-tale characteristic is the family's frozen state.

Once we thawed from our freeze and came to, realizing we were standing in front of a fast-moving bus, we were able to grab Cole and get to the side of the road. In our story, the side of the road was the safety of our hospital room where we were able to rely on others to get us through those first few days and make sure we were taking care of Cole and ourselves.

Nurses, child life specialists, doctors, family members, friends, our pastor, and many others shielded us on the side of the road and made sure the cancer bus didn't overtake and overwhelm us. The amount of support and guidance we received in those first few days and throughout treatment allowed us to progress through the shock and denial and do what we had to do to eliminate this cancer and get our son well again.

I believe it's important to provide information on the type of treatment Cole was about to receive since each type and stage of cancer receives a different arsenal of poison. Now, I am not a medical professional, so I feel it is important to focus on our experience and specific plan of treatment with the disclaimer that all experiences vary and treatment is different depending on the diagnosis, sub-type, and risk when it comes to leukemia.

Cole was diagnosed with T-cell acute lymphoblastic leukemia, so I am most familiar with this treatment protocol and the similar protocol of B-cell acute lymphoblastic leukemia. The drug names that coursed through my child's veins are forever embedded in my brain. Vincristine, methotrexate, PEG-asparaginase, Erwinase®, the cousins doxorubicin and daunorubicin, and cytarabine are only a few varieties in the poison cocktail my son would receive throughout treatment.

I memorized the protocol and the number of days and stages of each phase. Cole was placed on a high-risk protocol due to his age and white blood count at diagnosis. I won't inundate you with the different risk categories and subtypes, however, I will describe the steps of treatment Cole endured. He went through Induction, Consolidation, Interim Maintenance, Delayed Intensification, and Maintenance.

Two days after diagnosis, still in the PICU, induction began. The first chemotherapy put through his port was given by two amazing nurses whom we would encounter many times during our journey. These angels worked on Children's Three, the hematology/oncology floor and since the only inpatient nurses certified to give chemo were on the oncology floor and in clinic on the other side of the hospital, they came downstairs to the PICU to administer the red poison, daunorubicin, often nicknamed the "red devil" due to its color, potency, and potential side effects. This chemo was likely the most potent drug we encountered along with its cousin doxorubicin. To describe just how toxic this drug can be, researchers and medical professionals collaborated to establish a lifetime limit one person can receive.

There is a limit on the amount of red poison that can be administered to each patient based on many different factors. We were warned about the side effects which all sounded awful. However, one in particular stood out in my mind. Heart complications. This red poison that was going to kill the cancer running through my son's blood could cause issues with his heart. The heart that pumped his blood throughout his body, allowed him to play football and partake in other sports which also ran through his veins. For this reason, the limit was written into policies and strictly followed.

As I later learned, leukemia patients receive a small amount of this drug in comparison to other cancer patients, but precautions are still followed like an echocardiogram prior to treatment, one at the end of treatment, and one every five years for the rest of the patient's life to monitor any changes and intervene immediately. Even though the amount of poison is less than in other cancer protocols, heart complications can still occur so regular testing is necessary.

Yep, that seems like initiation by fire, right? Everything became real very quickly regarding the seriousness of these drugs when the nurses came into the room wearing blue suits, gloves, masks, eye protection and even the toxic chemical itself was wrapped in brown colored plastic to prevent any light from entering the iv bag while also hiding the red color of this devil. We never saw its face, just the after effects of nausea and red urine. We were warned about that one. I specifically remember the doctors and nurses saying not to freak out if Cole pees red because due to the coloring of the chemo, this was bound to happen.

The red devil, along with the escalating dose of methotrexate he received later in treatment, were the two drugs that caused the most nausea and vomiting. When I look back to the beginning of treatment, I realize how nervous this must have made Cole feel. The very first infusion he received is responsible for heart problems, pee the color of blood, and vomiting. I hope we did a good job of encouraging him and easing his mind as he was pummeled with side effects from the beginning.

A few days into treatment, I can't remember exactly when, but I do remember we were on Children's Three by that point so it was definitely day five or later, the steroids started to rear their ugly head. The hunger came like a raging beast and Cole began to crave specific things. Too bad he was still on a special diet due to his high potassium which made it extremely difficult to satisfy his junk food cravings.

Who would have thought potatoes contain a decent amount of potassium? Chips were definitely off limits as were multiple other favorites. When Cole was finally able to eat anything he wanted, his nurse who was one of the nurses who came to PICU to give Cole his first chemo, asked him what he wanted to eat now that he had free reign.

Cole's answer was a donut. Ok. I set off in search of the coveted pastry covered in rich chocolate icing and strategically placed sprinkles all in a perfect round shape. I feel like donuts are a pretty common, quick, breakfast item so it shouldn't be too hard to find, right? I walked every inch of the hospital, from the coffee cart out front, to the little coffee café, the atrium café, and a little convenience store type area. Nothing. Not one thing that resembled a donut anywhere in the building.

A few years prior, the hospital went all health food based and did an overhaul on everything offered throughout the building, even the gift shops. Finding a soda that was not diet was impossible, as well as any real chips or baked goods. If you like beet chips, vegetable chips, chickpea puffs or anything with vegetables and no sugar or taste, the options were unlimited. If you were a 14-year-old kid on steroids who just got off a super restrictive diet and craved salty and sweet, there were little to no viable options.

Since neither my husband nor I wanted to leave Cole's side for more than a minute or two, going out to get a donut was out of the question. My cousin offered to bring them on her next shift in the morning, but our amazing nurse overheard the conversation and by talking to Cole, found out the type of donuts he wanted. She approached a coworker coming in for the evening shift and literally an hour after Cole asked for them, there they were, a dozen of the gooiest, chocolate-covered, jelly-filled, powered, and Bavarian cream stuffed little circles of joy.

I never cried over donuts before. That was the first and only time since.

The compassion this nurse showed and the determination to get Cole the one thing he asked for while enduring a painful and draining few days in the hospital was heart-warming. I later asked her why she did it. This seemed like something way above and beyond her job duties and she said something like, "I was able to do it and it was important to Cole".

Simple acts of kindness like this meant more to our entire family than imaginable. Since we were no longer able to do routine things like leave the confines of the hospital and go to a donut shop, when others recognized this and stepped in, we were filled with joy and gratitude. Our nurse empathized with our situation and immediately sprang into action, making a child smile while devouring a chocolate donut.

For the last week, I had this nagging feeling that I was supposed to write about our hospital stay in general and the feelings that accompanied our initiation into the club that no one ever wants to be a part of, and those who have a membership would give it back in a second. I realize as I am typing these words, today is January 15th, the anniversary of Cole's diagnosis.

For the past three years, we have been members of this cancer club and will always be due to our experience. The feelings I am having while writing these words are so real that I can see myself in the hospital with Cole, going through the motions, not knowing what our journey would hold in the next months and years.

Even as I write our experience, I don't know what is going to happen in the future. No one does. This is the sole reason I always say "One Day at a Time". Don't look back. Don't look forward. Just be in the present moment and take it one minute at a time if you need. Keep going until the minutes add up to hours and the hours to days and days to weeks and so on. You just keep going, one step at a time.

Being admitted to the hospital holds a multitude of feelings. On the one hand, it was a busy place with lots of activity and we never felt alone. Even though things were difficult, Cole was very sick, and we weren't sure what was going to happen in the future.

There were people comforting us, talking to us, visiting, bringing things, and showing their support everywhere we turned. It felt almost like a hotel with lots of people, a gift shop, a cafeteria and anything else you could need. A very sterile, institution-style hotel with sick adults and children on every floor.

The hospital also felt safe in a way. I knew that if anything happened, there was a hallway full of nurses and doctors to help. I knew we could call someone and a moment later they would be in the room and know what to do. I was also still in shock due to how quickly things progressed and eternally grateful for the shock which propelled me through the long days and longer nights.

When we arrived home after being discharged, we reached a point of heightened anxiety because we were so used to having everything solved immediately and now if Cole didn't feel well or experienced a side effect, I had to call and wait to hear from someone with further instructions. The solution was no longer communicated instantly. There was what I call "the wait".

There was a sense of safety and calmness having Cole, my husband and me in one room in the hospital without distractions or responsibilities. We could focus all our attention on Cole and what he needed at that particular moment.

The first five days in the hospital were spent in the PICU. In the back of my mind, I knew my child was extremely sick. However, I also knew that nurses and doctors were watching him constantly, monitoring every breath, heartbeat, and blood level. The near constant care eased my mind and helped us support Cole in those first few days.

I never let my mind entertain the reason why we were placed in PICU. Literally, something could go wrong at any moment and having the staff and tools right there immediately was necessary. I still don't let my mind wander to the seriousness of Cole's illness or entertain the what-ifs that try to creep into my mind. I knew God was with us and would continue to be with us giving our family what we needed in the perfect time.

Not only did we have very capable hands caring for our child, but we also had family and friends praying for us and supporting us along the way. One of my very good friends who worked in our treating hospital for over a decade, came to the PICU when Cole was admitted. I mentioned a grief counselor I encountered in a previous role and continue to mention Mary Tiffin a few times in the book. This woman is an angel on Earth and has the quietest, most gentle grace about her that can put a person at ease even in the hardest of times. Mary took my hand and led me to an empty room and explained what was going to happen in the next few days and what to expect when Cole started treatment.

She wrote everything down in case it was overwhelming and when I couldn't remember her words, I had the notebook to reference when I needed a reminder of her wisdom. I still have her words and pictures written on the pages of that notebook, three years later.

Two analogies Mary used to describe what we were about to endure still stick out in my mind. I had no idea that leukemia treatment was over three years and my heart sank at the prospect of having to do this for over three years. How was I ever going to make it three months, let alone three years? As I re-read that statement, I have feelings of guilt and disgust.

If I was worried about making it over three years of treatment, how do I think my son felt? He was missing three pivotal years of school, friends, football, and normal teen life stuff. How dare I be worried about my emotional state. I would do whatever I had to do to support my son the best way I knew how so that he had the least number of emotional scars.

After I got over the shock of the length of treatment, Mary described what we were about to encounter as a roller coaster. Ups and downs, which even with my limited knowledge of cancer treatment, I knew this was to be expected. There would be good days and bad days, right? Got it. Nope.

What Mary explained was that yes, there were highs and lows, but the highs were extremely high, like the tallest roller coaster you have ever seen. Almost like you were on top of the world and everything was going perfectly fine. But the lows, the lows are super low. The bottom of huge coaster drops into that pit of bones in the Lion King where Simba and Nala get chased by the hyenas. That desolate land is what the lows of treatment resemble. From our experience, when the lows happen, there was despair, lots of prayers, questions to God about why this was happening, and feeling like nothing was ever going to turn around.

Eventually, we began to climb out of the desolate animal bone pit and see the sun once again. Every time was so awful and when we couldn't take any more stress or heartbreak, we saw the pathway to the exit of our desperation and the sun peeking behind a pile of bones indicating an easier journey ahead.

In the Lion King story, there were many ups and downs for Simba. From losing his father in a horrific accident, being tricked by his Uncle Scar and chased by hyenas who attempted to murder him, making sure he could not become king, to the point when his story turns around when he is rescued by two very unlikely creatures, discovered by an old friend, and eventually returns to his home, taking his rightful throne and restoring order to the pride.

In our story, there were many ups and downs as well. I started by describing our happy end of treatment celebration because we certainly understand that pediatric cancer is a dark, sad, and sometimes traumatic journey and difficult to read, let along walk the journey yourself. Then we return to chronological order with our diagnosis story and the shock that ran through our family, which was an extremely traumatic event that felt hopeless. We then moved through the first days of treatment in the hospital, which were also uncertain. But, in their uncertainty, those days gave us rest, and the ability to prepare for the journey ahead.

The highs occurred when it felt like everything was going right. Cole's counts recovered quickly, he didn't have a side effect of his medication, he didn't lose all his hair. When the highs occurred, we felt like we were on top of the world. I could see myself on the top of the roller coaster in an amusement park near our home where the flag sits signifying the high part of the ride. I felt unstoppable, relieved, and relaxed but I was also on edge and nervous because I knew the probability of things staying this way were slim to none.

During the difficult parts of treatment, this sentiment was like clockwork. No sooner did I get to the flag at the top of the hill than I was plummeting down to the bottom in the roller coaster car with my entire family along for the ride. Starting new things can be scary, especially when they involve super scary things like cancer.

Personally, I took solace in the support I received from family and friends. Knowing I was not alone in this journey gave me a sense of comfort and strength. Being in the hospital the first days of treatment, relying on the medical staff, receiving visits, prayers, comforting gifts and words of support helped me push through for my son.

I wasn't the one receiving treatment, enduring all the tests, being poked and prodded, sick and in the hospital, but I was there and all I could do was watch. It's heartbreaking, but I couldn't let my heart break. Holding it together for Cole took all my strength and power. I needed to replenish my strength from anywhere I could find it and give it to my son. We were at the beginning of something scary, but we had to keep moving to get to the calm and happy experience of ringing the bell at the end of treatment.

Now, I mentioned that Mary used two analogies to describe what we were going to go through during the course of treatment. The first, a roller coaster with extreme highs and lows, and the second was PAC-MAN.

You know, the little yellow guy on the screen of arcade games immortalized in the 1980s and still popular today? Well, if you have played or watched someone play PAC-MAN, you know that he eats everything in his path. Good and Bad depending on how savvy you are at navigating the yellow dot through the maze while being chased by bad guys.

Well Mary described chemo in the same way. Imagine chemo is PAC-MAN, eating everything in its way while being chased and threatened by cancer represented by the ghost-like objects trying to eat him and take over the body illustrated by the maze full of dots representing the cells. PAC-MAN doesn't have the time and knowledge to distinguish between the good and bad cells because he is being actively chased. So, what does he do? He eats them all.

This is how chemo works. Chemotherapy destroys all cells, good and bad, in hopes that the body can reset itself and continue fresh without the threat of cancer chasing and threatening to overtake everything. Hair, skin, nails, and even eyelashes and eyebrows are good, living cells but can be threatened and destroyed by the chemo. Living cells, like examples in the previous sentence, can be killed by the chemo in attempts to save the body (and ultimately the person) as a whole.

I get it now. Hair is a living cell and since PAC-MAN (or chemo) can't recognize that it's a good cell, not a bad cell, he eats it and hair falls out. It's pretty complicated because only certain types of chemo cause certain side effects just like certain players are extremely good at navigating and differentiating between the dots on the screen and others are novice players, rudimentary in their skills.

Having the analogies of a roller coaster to describe emotions during treatment and PAC-MAN to give chemo a face and describe its purpose helped us to understand things that were happening in our own language until we became fluent in cancer speak.

I touched on the first time Cole experienced chemo in the PICU, but he would get many more infusions during the first hospital stay, and in the years to come. Treatment itself consisted of round after round of poison and scheduled spinal taps where chemo was administered directly into his spinal fluid, so the cancer did not infiltrate this sacred space.

Fortunately, there were no cancer cells present in Cole's spinal fluid (CNS) at diagnosis, so he did not require radiation as part of his treatment plan. The spinal taps were done both as a diagnostic tool and preventative measure to ensure the cancer was kept at bay.

I realize that the beginning of our journey and the initial hospitalization and treatment overlap. Due to the progression of the leukemia and the results of the first bone marrow aspiration which indicated the percentage of leukemic cells in his marrow were 100%, treatment and diagnosis happened simultaneously.

In addition to diagnostic tests, beginning of treatment tests, managing symptoms Cole was already experiencing from dealing with the untreated cancer up until this point, and trying to support Cole's body and move it into a state where he gained enough strength for the battle to come, the battle had already started, and we didn't get a chance to rest before the fight. A blessing in disguise, the rapid pace in which everything occurred, allowed us to actively know we were treating Cole immediately to have the most favorable outcome.

The first few weeks of treatment held several purposes - kill the cancer, help Cole regain his strength, and prepare his body and mind for the long road ahead.

Cole

At the beginning of treatment, I was very overwhelmed. I was going to have to spend a large amount of time in the hospital. Everything in my life revolved around my diagnosis, chemo, appointments, and side effects. I went from not being in a hospital at all, to being there every day.

Treatment for my type of leukemia, T-ALL, is over three and a half years long. I thought at the most it would be a couple of months. I never thought it would be years that I would have to get chemo regularly. That's overwhelming to think about, having to do years of treatment. Before I started, I heard about how nasty chemo is in movies, TV shows, and the news, but I never experienced it myself or even had anyone in my family go through it, so I had no clue what to expect.

The first time I got chemo, I was still in the hospital. One of my favorite nurses, Bree, came down to the PICU with another nurse to give me my first dose. It was a really nasty, red chemo called daunorubicin. My oncologist told me they call this chemo "the red devil" because of its strength, color, and possible severe side effects. They even limit the amount of this you can have in your life because it can cause some bad things to happen to your heart.

I was already nervous to get chemo in the first place because of all the side effects I knew of like being nauseous and losing your hair, but this overwhelmed me even more because of what everyone was saying about it before it even started.

Getting the chemo the first time wasn't too bad because my port was already accessed. When I was in the hospital, they kept the needle in my port with a protective dressing over the top of it to make sure no germs got in that could cause infection. I couldn't really feel the needle in my chest at all. Although, I just received surgery to place the port so my chest was pretty sore since I didn't have time to recover before starting treatments. I was grateful for the port because I didn't have to get poked each time I needed chemo, and they could take blood right from my port which was already accessed every night so I didn't need to get stuck as much for blood counts.

The first time I got chemo, I did get nauseous. I was so puffy from all the fluids and pretty uncomfortable. I threw up a couple of times those first days of treatment. When I was finally allowed to go up to the third floor in the hospital, it felt good to be disconnected from the blood pressure cuff and the fluids were decreased too. Finally, I was free of all the wires and monitors but still had to take my IV pole with me wherever I went. I tried to go for walks a lot down the hallway and through the hospital because I felt pretty good, and it was boring being stuck in the room. The more I moved around, the better I felt.

A couple of days after the first chemo, I got another scary drug called PEG-asparaginase. My oncologist and my nurses told me that some patients reacted to his drug and I should tell them right away if anything felt weird. I wasn't super scared because I knew everyone was watching me and would help me if anything happened, but I was nervous about getting this chemo because it could cause me to not be able to breathe, so that was super scary.

The first couple of times I got it, I felt fine. My mouth did tingle and go a little numb, but my breathing was fine so I thought I would be ok. I was wrong. I'll talk about this in the next chapter, but I did have a scary reaction to the PEG and starting throwing up. I couldn't breathe, and I felt really weak. I remember grabbing onto my mom and yelling for her to help me. The next thing I remember is my nurse, Denise, stabbing my leg with something.

She told me later that it was an EPIPEN® that they used for allergic reactions to open my airway and help me breathe. I felt better a few hours later, but they told me I couldn't get that chemo again, and the chemo to replace it was in short supply so it might be hard to find.

I had only been in chemo for a couple of months at this point, so hearing they might not be able to find an important chemo made me nervous. My mom took care of everything and fought really hard to find it for me. She and another cancer mom, Laura Bray, worked together with the hospital and found all my medicine. I am proud of her for fighting so hard for me and finding a way so I didn't have to worry about it and could think about getting better.

The hard thing about the backup chemo was that I needed to get shots in my legs, and I couldn't just get it in an IV. The IV was so much better because I didn't even feel my port being accessed due to the numbing cream I used on my chest and my nurse, Barbie, was so good at accessing ports.

With the shots, the numbing cream didn't help at all. The only thing that dulled the pain was ice and that didn't even help decrease the burning sensation. The shots I needed burned so badly going into my legs, it felt like they were holding my legs in a fire. Afterwards, it made my legs hurt bad for days. The fact that I needed two shots every other day for two weeks didn't help either. My legs stayed sore the entire time and just started to feel better when the next round was about to start.

Another part of treatment that was difficult were the spinal taps. I got more in the beginning, but in maintenance I still got them every three months. I didn't feel anything during the spinal taps with chemo injected into my spine because I was asleep, but sometimes the next day I got spinal headaches which were awful. Nothing helped the headaches except lying flat and sometimes they lasted a week.

I was always pretty nervous when I got a spinal tap because I never knew if I was going to get a headache. Drinking a lot and even drinking caffeine right afterwards sometimes helped so I did this every time.

The first couple of times I needed to be put to sleep for the taps I was nervous. I had never been put under before my diagnosis, so I was afraid I wouldn't wake up. After a few times, I ended up getting used to it and liked how relaxed it made me feel before a serious procedure. My child life specialist, Rose, helped me a lot too because she was in the pediatric sedation area before she started in the clinic. She always talked to me about video games and distracted me by telling me she was going to mess with my hair. I still have all the hair stuff she used, and she made me laugh when I woke up and saw what she did.

Starting chemo was hard because it was so scary. I didn't know what to expect and I was really worried about losing my hair. My hair was super important to me and one of my best features, so I didn't want to lose it. My doctors, nurses, child life specialist, friends and family helped to calm me and get me ready for all the treatments. I knew treatment was the only option to get better, so I pushed through because I wanted to finally feel better and get back to feeling normal again.

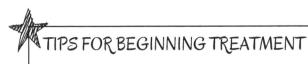

<u>Parents/Caregivers</u>

Take it one day at a time.

Just like during initial diagnosis, I suggest focusing on the present and take it moment-by-moment. If you can't focus on a whole day at a time, take it one hour at a time and increase the time until the days and weeks pass.

Take care of yourself. Yes, this is the last thing we think of, but it's necessary. You can't take care of your child if you are not in a good place personally. Make small goals and utilize resources (support groups, social worker, outside nonprofits). I found that just getting myself out of the hospital for a few minutes worked wonders.

Write things down.

You are going to receive an overload of information. I was not able to remember anything due to my state of shock. So, I found if I wrote things down and kept a binder, I was able to reference the information at any time.

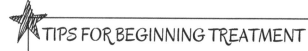

TIPS FOR BEGINNING TREATMENT

<u>Supporters</u>

Give the family grace. Realize they are going through something unimaginable and deserve all the prayers, space, forgiveness, grace, or support they need at that moment.

Understand their focus is on their child and will not be on work, friends, family, other obligations or activities.

Provide your support by offering to listen or help in any way needed. Don't pretend to understand what the family is going through because unless you walked in the same exact shoes, you can't.

CHAPTER 4

Treatment

In what was our new reality, we were forced to treat poison with poison, hoping the "good" poison would eradicate the bad poison (cancer).

Laura

Obviously, Cole's treatment journey has a lot of moving pieces, poisons, and places. The entire duration of his treatment did not occur during the initial hospital stay, nor did it occur solely during the first four weeks of induction. The clinic setting became our home away from home and thank goodness we lived close to the hospital because we really did spend most of our days in the stifling clinic rooms.

When Cole was discharged after 10 days in the hospital, it was our first victory. I will never forget Cole's face as he walked out of the hospital and saw the sunshine for the first time in almost two weeks. The glow illuminating from his body made me stop and take a breath, feel the gratitude of a simple sunshine, and the sun on my skin. Never would I let another moment be taken for granted because now our family knew just how precious these seemingly simple moments are and how quickly they can be taken away. At this specific moment in time, I realized you needed to lose just about everything to appreciate the joy in every moment.

We had a long road in front of us immediately after the initial diagnosis, but I learned in the very beginning to take everything "one day at a time". In the hard, unbearable moments, sometimes I needed to back it up to just one minute or one hour at a time, but I learned how to live in that exact moment. Limiting my focus to the task at hand helped to decrease the amount of information and anxiety getting into my system.

Since so much was happening at once and without warning, my brain did not have the capacity to look ahead or behind. I could only live in that particular moment in time and focus on the current task at hand. I've since realized that I often don't live in the moment when things are going well. I don't think about and appreciate the everyday things that occur, and I feel like I'm constantly dreaming about the future and how to make my life better even though it may be going well at the moment. When there isn't a traumatic event or important task occupying my attention, it's easy for my mind to become discontent with my current life situation. Going through such a traumatic experience allowed me to appreciate my life, be content with everything I have accomplished and cease comparing myself to others or wishing for different circumstances.

Coming face-to-face with your child's life-threatening illness puts everything into perspective in a very real way. No longer do the little mistakes or annoyances cause a catastrophe and the little things that we often take for granted have become the big things that I notice and remain grateful for at every turn.

Living in a time which has not yet occurred steals from the present. Treatment taught me to live in the present, enjoy the everyday blessings, and never take for granted one single moment because every moment we get on this earth is time we should not waste.

Throughout what we refer to as frontline treatment, which is the intense chemotherapy that lasts about nine months, our days consisted of long infusions at the clinic with the wait for chemo often being hours. The days started before 8 AM and usually didn't end until after 2 PM if not later.

Induction was the first round in the treatment journey and consisted of some potent poison to knock the white blood cell count down and get Cole into remission. Typically, leukemia patients will enter remission after induction. Although remission or MRD negative is achieved, which means a minimal residual disease of less than a certain percentage, there is no guarantee the patient will have such a favorable response to chemo.

If the patient does enter remission by achieving MRD negative status there is still no guarantee against a reoccurrence or negative side-effect to the chemo responsible for keeping the cancer at bay. Even though no cancer cells are detected by tests, there is always a possibility something can be there lurking around the corner or hidden out of view. For this reason, treatment continues for over three years total (for boys) to kill any cells they can't see and keep them from returning.

For four weeks, we woke up before seven in the morning and went to appointment after appointment for chemo and bloodwork, sometimes spending the entire day in the hospital. The type of poison pumped through his veins depended on the day and there were a few blood and platelet infusions thrown in the mix. At the end of induction, the real test arrived.

Cole had a bone marrow aspiration to check for MRD and a dose of intrathecal chemo (directly in the spinal fluid). The results would possibly declare him in remission on February, 14, 2020.

The first bone marrow aspiration done during diagnosis stated that 100% of the cells in Cole's body were leukemic. Due to this result, Cole's oncologist believed it would take longer to reach remission. I remember him telling me Cole would most likely not achieve MRD negative status just yet and it would take longer because all his cells were leukemic just four weeks ago. I was still very hopeful, and prayed continuously during the days between the test and when the results were ready.

As I write the date, I realize there is a thing with birthdays on holidays in our family. Cole's birthday is Christmas Eve, Kaden's birthday is April Fool's Day, my birthday is St. Nicholas day, while Josh's sometimes falls on Labor Day. So, the fact that Cole's remission date is on Valentine's Day does not shock any of us. This day is very much a birthday, a new beginning, and a celebration.

A few days after the 14th, I believe it was the 16th or 17th, but I can't be certain, I received a call. Knowing the results would be coming in any day, my chest tightened when I noticed it was the hospital calling. Upon hearing our oncologist's voice on the other end of the line, I think I stopped breathing as I walked out to our breezeway for a quiet moment to talk.

Noisy dogs and kids often make it difficult to have a conversation without yelling and I wanted to concentrate on each word he was speaking. When he uttered the phrase MRD negative and said remission, I believe I yelled into the phone. I was so relieved and surprised because we had all prepared ourselves for a longer battle to remission. The doctor was equally amazed and said it was a great sign. Thank God the chemo was working. Milestone one: remission accomplished.

After the initial phase of induction and the milestone of remission, we moved to the next territory called consolidation. We spent a good 12-16 weeks here where Cole's bone marrow and blood counts were bombarded by chemo after chemo, including a combination of Cytoxan® and cytarabine which knocked his white blood cell counts to zero on several occasions.

During this point in the game, Cole needed to drink lots of fluids and get fluids possibly before and after the initial infusion of this poison. I kept telling him how hydrated he needed to be and if he was hydrated, it would cut at least an hour off of our clinic stay that day. So, Cole was on a mission. He drank all evening and into the morning. He showed up, peed in the cup, and low and behold he was hydrated enough to start immediately. The nurses and doctors were surprised because this rarely happened. Even though we started earlier than expected, I think the chemo took extra long to arrive that day. Figures.

After the initial infusions, we were to give Cole injections at home three days in a row. I had to give my child a shot. I didn't think there was a way I could inject chemo into my child. Thankfully, my stepdad, who was a retired physician's assistant, offered to come when he could and give Cole the shot. He dropped everything he was doing and made sure to lessen our anxiety and Cole's, knowing a professional was controlling the syringe.

There were, of course, a few times when Josh and I had to do it because he took a part-time job in medical sales and wasn't available. At this point, I was still working in the office which puts me at my first two weeks of the job, the only time I was in office before the COVID protocols were put in place. Josh was still off on family medical leave at this point until we could figure out a better schedule. My husband didn't like injecting the chemo because he worried too much regarding his technique and making sure he was correct.

Obviously, I didn't want to inject my child either. Thankfully, between my stepdad and Josh, there was only one day when I had to give Cole the chemo. There was also only one day when it wasn't done correctly. Guess when?

I prepared the area, put down the sterile sheet, got the poison from the depths of our refrigerator in its brown, plastic, sealed bag far away from our food and drinks and got ready. I prepared Cole's skin, made sure everything was sterile, prepared my own hands by washing, scrubbing, sanitizing, and gloving. Now was the time. I got the needle ready to puncture a small hole in my child, pinched his skin, placed the needle, released the skin and…. "Mom, something's dripping". Oh no. I immediately stopped and pulled out the needle.

Springing into action, I cleaned the chemo off Cole's skin, put a BAND-AID® over the puncture and called the clinic. I told them what happened. I was mortified. Not only did I mess up literally the only time I needed to do this, but I was responsible for a missed dose. When I spoke to the nurses in clinic, they reassured me it was ok. It was only a small amount.

I immediately called my friend Laura who also had to give her daughter these same chemo injections. I was telling her exactly what happened and how mortified I was that I screwed up. Then I had a thought. Maybe God or some heavenly angel above saw something wrong with this chemo or syringe and for that reason it squirted onto the floor instead of inside my child's body. There had to be some reason I couldn't see that this would go wrong.

My explanation came during our next clinic visit. The Nurse Practitioner who took care of all the details, appointments, medication, tests and pretty much all the comings and goings of the clinic informed me that no one checked his batch of needles which they do as a courtesy to make sure they are on the syringe tightly. Since an outside pharmacy prepares the chemo and the supplies needed to give the medication, the hospital can't guarantee anything but our nurse tries to double-check everything when they have the chance. She noticed a few needles in batches she was checking the past couple of days were loose and since we received this medication on her day off, that is most likely what happened to us. She explained they usually checked them, but don't always get the chance, and I should make sure to give it a good turn to make sure everything is secure the next time.

No, this didn't make me feel much better, but it did help explain what happened. I had to keep reminding myself I cannot control everything. I am not in control of how things happen and even though I do my best, things beyond my control can and will occur and I need to come to terms with this fact.

The toxic, one-two punch of this chemo combination caused Cole's counts to drop pretty low. Every single time the protocol reached this point, his numbers bottomed out and we put neutropenic protocols in place. Having low counts was anxiety inducing because literally any germ could infiltrate his non-existent immune system and send us to the hospital in a flurry. The threshold to measure immune system response was an ANC (absolute neutrophil count) of 500. Anything below this magic number meant there was virtually no immune system response and extreme measures needed to be taken to protect Cole from anything that could get him sick. This meant eating over cooked foods, no raw vegetables, no flowers in the house, no exposure to pets in our home, everyone wearing a mask and keeping sick people away.

When his ANC was above 500 but below 1,000, there was some immune system response, but not enough to lift the neutropenic protocols I just mentioned. The magic number that indicated we could let our guard down was 1,000. When we hit that magic number, Cole often indulged in a salad. Yes, a leafy green vegetable salad with meat and cheese was what he often craved, or a hoagie from Subway just beneath the clinic since lunch meat was also a member of the banned food list.

Cole and I spent a lot of time together in that small clinic room, waiting, talking, interacting with staff, and sometimes I sat in the uncomfortable chair with little leg room just watching his beaten body rest. For 10 months, thanks to chemo holds, a chemo shortage, and stubborn counts, this was our existence.

For a few months, we were at the clinic at least three times a week. The rare days off felt like a breath of fresh air or a weekend day after a long day of work. Besides seeing the poison drip into my child's veins and needle after needle go into his chest to access his port, watching him physically struggle was an absolutely heart-wrenching part of the journey.

From reading the past couple of chapters, you can already get a sense of the type of person Cole was before and after treatment. During the awful parts of treatment, he carried the same quietness, mental and physical determination, intelligence, and respect that he always possessed (and still does). Even when in extreme stress and pain, his face remained stoic, and he complied with every poke and prod with a strength that far surpasses my capabilities.

Treatment was tough. It had to be tough in order to kill the cancer that took over my child's body in a short amount of time. Along with the extremely long days, the hours of silence spent waiting for test results, medication or chemo and the emotional fatigue of such traumatic events day after day, Cole also had to deal with a variety of side effects from the poison meant to save his life. As if it weren't bad enough to have to live at the hospital when he was supposed to be at home doing virtual school due to COVID like everyone else, he was riddled with side effects and reactions that landed us hospitalized more than once.

The doctors, nurses and child life specialist became members of our family. We shared everything with them and they, in turn, with us. Day after day we spent hours with these amazing, intelligent and compassionate individuals. In this phase of our life, the majority of our time was spent within the walls of the hospital, usually in the pediatric oncology clinic.

Our hospital is small in comparison to hospitals in cities, but large for our area. The small town feel echoes in each hallway, office, clinic, and inpatient floor. Even in the valet, I was greeted by name each morning. Since there were about three valet drivers and we were using their services almost daily, it didn't take very long for them to remember my name.

One of these amazing employees would smile every time my big, gray, F150 pulled into the valet lane. Most days she would wave her hands like an air traffic controller, dance, or greet me with a loud "Laura, nice to see you". I always had a little conversation with her as we began our day, and it made us smile. Also, the woman at the valet checkout counter inside the hospital would always say hello and talk to us while we waited to leave at the end of our days. We always knew if it was an extra-long day by her comments "you were here a while today" or "it's pretty early, didn't take long today, huh?"

Sharing the past few years with the same employees who saw us at our worst and followed our journey to see the victories helped us on the bad days and made the good days even better.

Our nurses are no different. The clinic nurses changed a bit in the past three years, but each nurse is an important part of our story. Our BFF, the funniest and most outrageous nurse who knew when to calm my craziness or encourage my antics holds a special place in our hearts. Denise has been there through the bad and the good, calls Cole her BFF, and even came a few Christmases and birthdays to sing to Cole and bring him a gift. She is just silly enough to make a smile form on my teenager's face. The cupcake and fairy BAND-AIDs® she selected each time she took the needle out of Cole's chest and carefully covered the puncture were always over the top just like her.

Everyday Cole was offered snacks and drinks since we were literally there all day almost every day. He never asked for anything and rarely told them if he wanted a snack. Denise saw Cole's quiet, thoughtful, and sometimes embarrassed nature and realized he would never ask for anything. So, she always had special snacks waiting for Cole when we returned from a test or spinal tap, and she carefully picked out school-colored freeze pops during chemo.

I mentioned before that Cole played football and the sport was missed incredibly the three years he had treatment. Denise's son also played football, but for a different team. So, depending on the day, she would give him a red pop for Cole's school or a purple or orange colored pop for her son's school. Ever the quiet soul, Cole always shook his head and smiled while eating the grape or orange flavor. When our sweet nurse took a different job, we made sure to give her a little care package complete with a BFF necklace. To this day, Cole has half and Denise has the other half.

Several other nurses came and went, but one remained the same. A fixture of the hospital at this point with 40 plus years of experience all in the same clinic. An angel on this earth that has seen a great deal working with pediatric cancer patients and their families for such a long career. Hailing from my hometown about 35 minutes from the hospital and the mom of two children near my age who went to the same small, Catholic elementary school as I, her wisdom and compassion was a constant during our entire length of treatment.

Before we even got to the clinic, we heard that she was the best nurse to access ports and many patients wouldn't let anyone but her touch their chests with a needle. A tiny lady with a large personality and voice you could recognize just about anywhere, she became our lifeline during those long days at the hospital. Her name is just as iconic as she is and denotes her as a fixture, famous face, long-standing, and loyal employee who all the children know. Barbie has become a part of our family and many of the other families treated at the hospital.

Having the best team behind us as we marched forward on our journey was imperative. As I have mentioned many times, cancer is hard, but chemo is nasty. In order to rid Cole's body of the cancer cells and retrain it to produce healthy cells, we needed to kill off the bad cells for good.

Currently, there is no way to just aim at the bad cells. So, many good cells got taken down as well. Remember the PAC-MAN analogy? He eats everything, good and bad. As if this way of treatment isn't bad enough in and of itself, the side effects of a nasty poison often cause more harm than the cancer itself.

Some patients get so sick from the side effects of the chemo or infections as a result of a weakened immune system, that it's not the cancer that causes problems. It's the chemo and its terrible nature to kill and destroy. Yes, the cancer is awful and made Cole very sick, but the treatment used to cure his body and rid him of illness also caused terrible days and a few hospital admissions along the way.

Cole

I talked a little bit about treatment and how it started but most of the treatment wasn't while I was admitted in the hospital. They had an oncology clinic and I spent almost every day there. I'm glad we lived close to the hospital because these were already really long days, and a long drive would have made it a lot longer.

I had nine or 10 months of hard chemo and then around two years of maintenance chemo because I was allowed to end treatment a couple of months early. During the first nine months, I was at the clinic a lot after I got out of the hospital. Even though I wasn't in the hospital, I still had to go almost every day and they often lasted the entire day from seven in the morning until two or three in the afternoon, sometimes later.

We waited in the waiting room in the clinic until a nurse came for me. They always checked my height and weight because the chemo was based on my weight. They needed to be exact. After my weight was checked, my temperature and blood pressure were checked, too. I was taken to a room, and it was usually the same room, number five. My nurse, Denise, always called it the "Cole Suite". It was one of the only rooms with a normal sized chair.

The exam tables were too small, so I liked to sit in the chair to get chemo. It's really the only place I was kind of comfortable. Each clinic visit started the same. The nurses asked a bunch of questions and ran through all my medications, making sure I was taking everything and to see if I had any problems with the treatment.

My port was accessed almost every time I went to the clinic. I put a numbing cream on the spot at home and that helped a lot. I don't like the way a lot of things feel against my skin, so it took me awhile to find the right BAND-AID® to seal in the cream. My nurses wanted me to use press and seal which is a plastic wrap, but I didn't like the way it felt. The tricky thing was that the chemo made my skin super sensitive so any type of adhesive on my skin blistered and turned red. The nurses had to use a special covering for my port when it was accessed so my skin didn't get irritated. In the beginning, they didn't know how sensitive my skin actually was, so the regular dressing was used. My skin got so raw and red and even bubbled. As soon as the nurses noticed, they switched to a special dressing for sensitive skin. Apparently, this was pretty common. In addition to the normal side effects of each chemo, skin sensitivity often happened as well.

The days at the clinic were often long because I needed to get blood counts almost every time to make sure my levels were ok to get chemo. Sometimes we waited for hours for the counts to come back. If my counts were low, I needed platelets or blood, and that took even longer. I don't even know how many transfusions I got during treatment, but it was definitely more than 20.

Sometimes I didn't make counts and then I was placed on a chemo hold which meant I didn't get the chemo until my counts reached the number they needed to start again. This happened a couple of times towards the end of the hard stage because my bone marrow was beat up so much from the hard chemo over the last few months that it took longer to bounce back. The doctors said this was normal and often happened during certain stages.

If my counts were ok, then I got the chemo which was another wait. There was only one chemo pharmacy in the hospital and sometimes it took a while. Getting the actual chemo took anywhere between 20 minutes and an hour, which was definitely the shortest part of the day.

When the chemo was done, I got de-accessed (the needle was taken out of my chest) and a BAND-AID® was put over my port. My nurses always gave me the funniest BAND-AIDs® and they made me smile.

My entire life revolved around chemo and going to the hospital. There was a lot of waiting, which was the hardest part. I wanted to be home and resting, but instead, I was in a little room waiting for medicine. I wish they could give you chemo in your own home, which would be a lot more comfortable. I used to wish they actually did that, but I understand it's not possible. So, we went to the clinic multiple times a week. It was better than staying in the hospital.

The hardest chemo was in the beginning. I did induction for one month and then got a spinal tap to check if I was in remission. I was so happy to get the results that I was, indeed, in remission and the chemo was working. It was actually Valentine's Day when I had the spinal tap and a couple of days later I found out I was in remission.

After induction was a couple of months of consolidation when my counts dropped pretty low and I also had a reaction to PEG and ended up in the hospital. I had a fever and was shaking so bad, like I had the flu. My mom took me straight to the ER and since it was right when COVID started, I needed to be taken to a sealed room and tested for COVID because I had a fever. We were isolated for at least a day, first in the ER and then in the PICU. We couldn't leave the room at all and even though I wasn't really sick, I still needed to keep a mask on in my sealed room. It was very uncomfortable. Once I found out the COVID test was negative, we went up to my normal floor of the hospital.

During this time, I didn't have a port because my port got infected. The first port never worked right and didn't heal, so when it developed a puffy bubble the nurses told my doctors right away. It was removed that same day and I was put on antibiotics just in case. I had to wait six weeks to get another port so that meant a lot of pokes. Before this time, I had pretty good veins but having to be poked multiple times a day every day for a week while I was in the hospital was a lot. I even had two IVs at one point. I remember telling my nurses that the one IV wasn't working right. They didn't use it, but didn't take it out either and I ended up with cellulitis, a skin infection and I was put on antibiotics again.

When I got my second port, I was happy because it worked great and healed a lot faster than the last port. Having the port in my chest made chemo so much easier because I didn't need an IV and the vein my port connected to was a lot bigger so it was less likely to damage.

When the first ten months or so were over, I entered the maintenance phase. During maintenance, chemo wasn't as often. The first three cycles of maintenance (each cycle was three months) I still needed to get nelarabine which I received during my frontline treatment. This particular chemo was given each day for five days in a row. The nurses kept my port accessed and covered it with a special dressing during that time, so I didn't have to get accessed every single day. Sometimes I chose to take a break from being accessed halfway through the five days but usually I just left the needle in place to make things easier.

Since I was accessed with a needle in my chest, I couldn't do any rough activities and had to be extra careful. I also couldn't run or do strenuous activities like play basketball because of a possible side effect with my muscles that could happen with this particular chemo.

I'm grateful this time was during COVID because I couldn't play basketball or go to the park with my friends anyway. Since no one was able to be with each other that made it a little easier and I didn't feel like I was missing so much.

Once the nelarabine was finished, which was nine months into maintenance, the only hard part of treatment remaining were the spinal taps. They were every three months and still caused headaches. During maintenance, my counts stayed around 1,000 so I could eat salads and didn't have to be as careful as when they were low. At this point, most things returned to normal. I only went for chemo once a month, but took pills every night at home. It was nice being back to normal for the most part. Things in the world were finally getting back to normal too, so I could do a lot more than when I was in active treatment and COVID was worse.

I was getting closer to having an even more normal life, without chemo and healing my body from the years of chemo and medication I needed day after day.

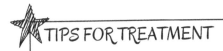

TIPS FOR TREATMENT

<u>Parents/Caregivers</u>
One treatment at a time.

They may all go differently so live in the present and take it one treatment at a time.

Ask questions.

Get as much info as you can.

Know what to watch for.

Call if you forget.

Keep all information/take notes.

Write down important things, but if you are unsure at any point, call the office.

Make a schedule on a calendar.

We used a white board calendar on our refrigerator to keep track of chemo days, medication doses, and other appointments. Use a pill organizer to keep track of steroids and chemo. Make sure you are still giving the medication directly to your child and make sure they are taking it in front of you. The organizer helped us keep track and make sure we didn't forget or double up on doses which could be awful.

CHAPTER 5

Side Effects

Chemo is a poison that cannot differentiate between good and bad cells. So, it kills both the good and the bad with the hope of starting over with completely new (and hopefully) healthy cells. The poison destroys everything in its path causing potentially serious side effects.

Laura

Have you ever heard the saying "stuck between a rock and a hard place"? It's often used to describe a situation where it's pretty much lose, lose.

I imagine this huge bolder that has me pinned up against a brick wall. I'm stuck. There is no moving that bolder and the brick wall sure isn't going to move and allow me to wiggle free. When facing a cancer diagnosis and hearing the options of treatment, some things like chemotherapy, lumbar puncture, surgery, or radiation may be discussed depending on the type and stage of cancer. All of these treatments carry risks. Not doing treatment is not an option.

So, we are faced with the fact that poison is going to be administered to kill the cancer. Even though we have advances in technology, doctors do not yet have the ability to target that poison at only the cancer cells, sparing the rest of the body from its effects. Sure, certain treatments like CAR T-cell therapy and immunotherapy are likely to be used widely as a targeted treatment approach, but the laser focus, precise treatment of only killing the cancer and sparing the rest of the body from its toxic effects, is not yet an option.

We are resigned to the fact that treatment can be less than pleasant on the body. More times than not, the treatment plan involves some type of chemo. According to the Mayo Clinic, since it was the first result of my Google search, "chemotherapy is a drug treatment that uses powerful chemicals to kill fast-growing cells in your body. Chemotherapy is most often used to treat cancer."

Right in the definition of chemotherapy, the expert writers are telling us that chemo is powerful. It is also mentioned that it's a chemical. I refer to it as a poison because it literally is a poison. It's powerful. It must be powerful to face an opponent like cancer. However, being so toxic and powerful does not come without the risks. I hate that the go-to options to fight cancer are toxic and can create destruction in our children's bodies.

So, in other words, what I am saying is that there was no choice in treatment options for Cole's particular type of leukemia. The current protocol for T-cell acute lymphoblastic leukemia has a high success rate and that is exactly what we want - success. There was no debating on the type of chemo Cole was going to receive or any other option of treatment than the Children's Oncology Group (COG) protocol which was the plan followed by our treating hospital and many other hospitals in the area.

We've had to make a lot of difficult and heart-wrenching decisions in the past three years, but deciding what type of poison to fight another poison with was not one.

There is solace in the fact that the plan was already mapped out with the exact doses, types, and way of administering. The plan puts my mind at ease knowing that we followed the treatment that worked and continues to work for so many patients. When we were in the thick of the fight, the toxic effects and possible long term side effects were always in the back of my mind, but did not come to the front begging for immediate attention because killing the cancer, going into remission, and improving Cole's overall health was absolutely urgent.

Now that Cole is off treatment, it pains me to look back and remember everything his teenage body endured. All the side effects are discussed before starting treatment and even before starting each new medication.

We received a sheet of medication information, just like the sheet you receive after getting a vaccine for yourself or your children. The medication is listed, the possible side effects, and situations in which you should call the doctor. Before even being discharged from the hospital, I had quite a large pile of these frightening informational pages.

One of the first medications Cole started was dexamethasone, a steroid. Not the anabolic kind of steroid that pumps up your muscles, but the kind of steroid that decreases inflammation and fights certain ailments like poison ivy or an allergic reaction. This tiny little pill packs a huge punch. It can cause sleeplessness, a round puffy moon shaped face, weight gain, insatiable hunger, and roid rage. Yep, that part is really true.

I remember a conversation with a mom whose daughter went to the same school as Cole and was diagnosed with cancer a year before Cole's diagnosis. I believe we were still admitted to the hospital at the time, so the medications and their effects were not embedded in my brain at this point. The mom was telling me her daughter had "roid rage" and that it was not some mythical occurrence. The mood swings often described when explaining what happens when you take steroids (usually describing the weightlifting, illegal stuff) are completely real.

Steroid week (not to be confused with "shark week") was always dreaded because the sleeplessness, moodiness, yelling, and crazy appetite were often hard to handle along with everything else treatment was throwing at us at that point in time.

Cole had two different kinds of steroids during treatment, dexamethasone and prednisone. Dexamethasone, often referred to as dex, was used during the intense portion of chemotherapy called frontline. Prednisone came into the game during the maintenance phase, benching the dex for good.

Cole reacted stronger to the dex than the prednisone. I know some protocols that use the prednisone in frontline and dex in maintenance. I also know some children who do better with dex than prednisone. Everyone is different and every situation varies.

Some of the side effects Cole experienced from steroids were: sleeplessness, itchiness, weight gain, a puffy moon shaped face, crazy hunger, weird cravings, rage and diabetes. Yep, diabetes.

One of the scarier side effects, the combination of the dex and Erwinase® which can both cause a rise in blood sugar, caused Cole's blood sugar to raise to almost 350.

Cole's high blood sugar was probably one of the scariest side effects we experienced and managed at home. Most of the other reactions mandated that we be admitted to the hospital but as I'll describe later, we were able to give insulin at home to manage this scary situation. Due to a drug shortage, one of Cole's medications was delayed. Due to this delay it was given in combination with the dexamethasone. Erwinase®, which can cause a rise in blood sugar (along with dex), caused Cole's blood sugar level to climb to around 350. This is almost three times the high end of the normal scale.

When the diabetic episodes started, we were more than halfway through the intense nine-ten months of chemo before maintenance was to begin. Usually the steroid and Erwinase® are not given simultaneously since they can cause similar side-effects, but it was necessary in our case, due to the drug shortage which resulted in an inability to secure the medication in time for his scheduled dosage.

Cole's diabetic episode presented by signs that he was extremely thirsty halfway through the steroid week, and was up all night drinking water like he couldn't get enough. Of course, he didn't wake either of us because Cole never wanted to bother us and usually suffered in silence (we are working on this). The next day, we went into the clinic for a scheduled appointment. When I mentioned this new symptom, his nurse was immediately concerned and asked the doctor if she could draw a little extra blood to test his sugar. The results were not completely surprising but just as devastating. A sugar of 350 was dangerous and needed to be treated with insulin.

Now, I was tasked with giving my 14-year-old insulin shots and monitoring his blood sugar throughout the day. I knew how to monitor blood sugar to a small extent because I had gestational diabetes toward the end of my pregnancy with Cole. I never needed insulin, so injecting my child in the back of the arms with an insulin pen multiple times a day was a new experience for both of us. Remember, the chemo injections did not go well for me, but this was different and a pen-like device instead of syringe.

The hospital has diabetes educators that come into the clinic room and teach you how to use the insulin and what to do if their sugar bottoms out and they are unresponsive which is an emergency situation, but it's imperative to be aware and be prepared should this occur.

I vividly remember our nurse telling us that she thought Cole would be admitted, and Cole immediately burst into tears. This, and an unexpected additional day to an already long admission were the only two times he became visibly upset. Cole is the strongest individual I have ever met, and I knew he was tired of being dealt a bad hand. By the grace of God, the endocrinologist entrusted with Cole's care, did not admit us that day. Her kind personality, intelligence and competency stood out immediately when we met her in clinic that day. She immediately established a positive rapport with Cole and I could tell because he became relaxed and at ease.

At this point, Cole had already been admitted twice beyond the initial, 10-day admission at diagnosis and he had enough. He could not catch a break and reaction after reaction and multiple side effects and nausea all seemed to happen at the same time. All we both wanted was to be able to go home that night and relax in our beds while watching TV and making ourselves comfortable in our own space, not a hard hospital bed with interruptions every few minutes.

So, saying it was a blessing that we were able to go home was an understatement. We left the clinic that day, armed with insulin, alcohol, needles, a meter, test strips, and the emergency glucagon. We were also given a paper that outlined how many units of insulin to give Cole depending on his blood sugar reading and instructions of what to do in an emergency.

A million questions were racing through my head upon arriving home. Was I going to be able to inject insulin into my child? Was this going to be permanent? Why were things so difficult? How was I supposed to act like everything was ok when it wasn't?

Those are just some of the thoughts and questions plaguing my mind and stealing any type of relaxation I thought I deserved.

So, I said a prayer and asked God to help me through this difficult time and give us the guidance we needed at that moment. I also asked Him to protect my son and restore his blood sugar to normal levels and then I called my friend, Laura. Her daughter was also in treatment for leukemia although she was almost finished at that point. Since they were ahead of us in the journey, I often called her when I was in despair.

If anyone could understand what I was facing, it was her. Several times during treatment, when I didn't think I could take one more thing happening, I reached out to a fellow cancer mom and was immediately understood. I knew that even if they didn't understand exactly what was going on or what was happening at that point in our journey, at least I wasn't alone.

In the silence and the solitude, my mind immediately attempted to convince me that we were facing this alone and we were the only family in the entire world in these dire circumstances at this moment. Terrifying and cruel, these were thoughts that entered my brain at the worst moments. I knew in my heart they weren't true, but I needed to find out for myself that others were with us in this battle. Having the support of family and friends was one thing that helped, but reaching out to other cancer moms hit a level of calm I usually couldn't reach. Extremely hard to explain, yet explainable with one word: understood.

The conversation I had with Laura while I was sitting on my front porch steps crying and doubting my ability to inflict more pain on my son in order to lower his sugar will forever be one of many moments in which I allowed myself to spill everything into someone else's heart and be supported, understood, and refilled.

Having this conversation allowed me to get up, dust myself off, and try again. Yes, that was an Aaliyah reference for those 1990s/early 2000s teens. I'll talk about Laura again in the pages to come because she has done way more amazing things for our family in addition to drying my tears and calming my crazy.

It will never be determined for sure, but since the Erwinase® had to be delayed due to the issue of not being able to secure the medication right away and the steroid and Erwinase® had to be given together, it could have caused the diabetic blood sugar levels. The good news was that after the medication was finished, there was a good likelihood that the blood sugar would return to normal. It turns out that each time Cole was put on dex, which was about once a month for about three more months, he did indeed have blood sugar issues. When Cole entered maintenance, Erwinase® was finished and the steroid was switched to prednisone, everything resolved.

I understand that Cole's blood sugar could have reached a dangerous level even if the Erwinase® was on time, but the fact that it happened when it did and there was a delay in the medication, pushes me to advocate for the timely arrival of live-saving medication and awareness of drug shortage issues. Because we experienced a drug shortage, I want to work with others to make sure that if anyone else is experiencing a shortage, they are not alone.

In addition to dangerous blood sugar levels and the need for insulin while receiving steroids, Cole reacted to the methotrexate. This drug is used widely in his treatment protocol, including being injected into his spinal fluid during his frequent spinal taps, also called lumbar punctures.

One of the major differences between the approach for B-cell and T-cell leukemias is that patients who have B-cell leukemia get a high dose methotrexate while the T-cell patients receive an escalating dose of the same drug. The high dose protocol requires hospitalization, fluids, and monitoring to make sure the drug leaves the body within a certain time. Cole did not require hospitalization and fluids because his dose was much lower.

Of course, Cole reacted to the methotrexate and did not metabolize it quickly, so it stayed in his body causing vomiting, dehydration, a skin rash, mucositis, and yeast-like open sores on his body. He couldn't swallow or move without excruciating pain. He was so nauseous that we ended up in the ER multiple times for fluids due to dehydration.

The last time he was in the ER, he was admitted due to the mucositis, not being able to keep anything down and the raw, open sores covering a good part of his body. The after effects of this medication were brutal. Cole could not even keep clothes on his body because it felt like daggers on his raw skin. Cole also has a condition called hidradenitis suppurativa. Well, apparently methotrexate can cause skin rashes and in turn made his hidradenitis super angry. It was a perfect storm creating a multitude of brutal skin reactions.

Open, festering and raw, these wounds live near sweat glands and often occur in the armpits and groin. Lucky Cole. Methotrexate made his skin so angry that he developed hidradenitis and yeast-like raw sores in these areas of his body. They were so incredibly painful that he couldn't move or change positions without being in complete agony.

I felt so hopeless when we got to the hospital because I didn't even know. I didn't know that my son had these sores all over his body until he was so tired and in so much pain from vomiting uncontrollably that I forced my hand and took him to be seen because he couldn't keep anything in his system. The skin reaction was still a mystery at this point. He was taking frequent showers, but I thought it was to ease the nausea. I had no idea the magnitude of the hardships this tough soul was experiencing.

Upon reaching the emergency department, I noticed little pimple like sores all over Cole's head. I pointed them out to the doctor, but he was more concerned with getting some fluids into my son and supporting his liver and kidneys. So, when we got to the inpatient floor, the nurses and doctors gave him a complete exam. That is when the horror came to light.

When the doctor raised his arms and looked at his legs, the true picture was seen. The absolute terror that reached out and grabbed ahold of me while standing next to my son was a combination of sadness, anger, and pity. "How could he keep this from me" was my response. I couldn't understand why Cole didn't tell me what was going on and I suddenly remembered the frequent showers he was taking the last couple days and the foul, green liquid that covered his armpit the previous day that I quickly stole a glimpse of before he noticed and immediately covered himself with his blanket.

After we were admitted, one of our favorite nurses, Joe, came on shift and saw Cole laying there with only a towel on. It hurt too much to even have fabric touch his raw skin. Our nurse just looked, laughed, and said "guess

we're not doing clothes today". That hospital admission was also the time
we met Bridget. She was a quiet, kind nurse on night shift who was the
only person that offered to get Cole ice for his sores, brought us a fan,
and helped Cole apply cream to his body every few hours.

To describe how big of a deal this is, you need to know the kind of
teenager Cole is. Cole is quiet, an introvert, shy and super intelligent. He is
the student in the classroom who knows all the answers to what the
teacher is asking, but never raises his hand. Cole is also the quiet, well-
behaved kid staying at a friend's house who would rather go hungry or
thirsty than ask for something to eat or drink.

Bridget saw this in Cole and instead of asking him and having the
automatic response of "no", she did not take no for an answer. She saw
he needed help, and literally dove right in helping him when he needed it
most.

In May of 2022, we had another unplanned admission and saw Bridget
again. This time, she was the charge nurse and came to greet us saying
"I'm a big girl, now". I was so proud in that moment to be able to see her
when she first started and was on shift with a mentor nurse to that
moment when she was a confident and respected nurse and leader.

We had many other experiences like this with people who have helped us.
Never ever judge a book by its cover. That quiet and introverted nurse
could have the biggest impact on your experience. Sure, we love the
outgoing and funny nurses, the confident and vocal leaders, but there is

something about people who do not fit the mold that often surprises us in such a good way.

In addition to the PEG-asparaginase anaphylactic reaction, the diabetes, methotrexate sores, allergic reactions to antibiotics, bandage adhesive and BAND-AID® reactions, and cellulitis due to a bad IV, Cole also experienced another rare reaction in May of 2022. Apparently, Cole was exposed to the Epstein-Barr virus (EBV) which is the virus that causes mono. This darn mono keeps popping up throughout our journey.

As a result of this exposure to his fragile immune system, the virus attacked his appendix. What Cole experienced is super rare in patients undergoing chemotherapy. In fact, our hospital doctors have only seen it in patients who previously had a transplant.

From what I understand, transplant patients are monitored for EBV detection monthly due to the possibility of potential EBV-related illnesses. Since anti-rejection medication keeps their immune system in a constant state of fragility the EBV can cause harm. Therefore, monthly blood tests to detect the virus are necessary to ensure treatment happens immediately and little damage is done.

The doctor explained to us that EBV can do one of two things when it affects the system of an immunocompromised individual. It can "peeve off" some area of the body, which in Cole's case was his appendix, or it can mutate and affect the lymph nodes and cause a type of lymphoma called Burkitt lymphoma which is a type of non-Hodgkin lymphoma.

This happens when the EBV causes the lymphocytes in the blood which are partly responsible for fighting infection to divide like crazy instead of fighting the infection (EBV) like usual. The doctors were unsure of which category Cole's reaction fit, but they were leaning toward the first, with the appendix listed as a casualty.

Cole's doctors were pretty sure his reaction fell into the category of the infection-fighting blood cells attacking his appendix because they believed it was a threat. Due to his suppressed immune system, it could not pinpoint the actual threat and attacked his organ instead. This is super complicated and made my head spin. It's also extremely rare; of course. We needed to complete some more tests including blood tests and CT scans. If the EBV was detected throughout his body we needed to start immunotherapy immediately to calm down the response of the cells and re-direct them into fighting the virus and not his healthy organs and cells.

We just went through a really tough week of an admission, a ruptured appendix, emergency surgery, extreme pain, and a slow recovery process and then we were hit with the fact that Cole's appendix tested positive for EBV. Right when we thought we were on the road to recovery, an unseen player came onto the field and tackled us, pushing us to the sidelines and causing us to take a pause in the game to treat the injuries this mysterious opponent caused.

The actual reaction started with a sore side. Cole had extreme pain in his right, lower side area. He was throwing in track and field at the time, so he originally thought he pulled a muscle in his side. The day we ended up in the emergency room, his pain was so bad at school that he couldn't stand upright without grasping his side. Cole, being the strong person that he is, did not want to go to the hospital and tried extremely hard to brush it off. That evening, he developed a 102-degree fever which made the decision easy due to his port. We were going to the hospital.

Because Cole had a mediport in his chest, anytime there was a fever of at least 101, we were instructed to take his temperature again in an hour and if it was still high, we needed to head to the emergency room. Since his fever was 102, we didn't need to wait. We could head right into the ER.

Initially the doctor in the emergency department didn't think Cole's appendix was in jeopardy because he didn't have the usual symptoms of extreme stomach pain, vomiting, or other stomach issues. An ultrasound of his abdomen showed something was not quite right with his colon or intestines, but the tech couldn't find his appendix because it's a tiny, hidden organ that is difficult to see in ultrasounds.

A surgeon was called and came into our little, sealed room to explain that it looked like his colon was growing into itself and they were going to do a CT scan so they could see more clearly. Usually, this phenomime occurs in much younger children and the symptoms didn't align. So, they needed to do more testing. I was super confused and anxious, thinking we had a whole separate battle on our hands and possibly a risky surgery. I didn't know what to think at this point but something in the back of my mind told me we would be ok and this was a mistake. By doing the CT scan, I believed they would figure out exactly what was going on.

After the CT was performed, the appendix was seen and the diagnosis was a definitive appendicitis. The surgeons never really talked about the colon until after the surgery was complete. From what was seen on the scan, it appeared to be a normal appendicitis and not ruptured.

Knowing what we were dealing with was both a relief and a curse. I felt relieved that we didn't have this super complicated surgery to go through because it was a routine appendicitis, but we also had to go through another surgery and hospital stay with a few weeks recovery time when Cole was finally at the point in treatment when he was returning to a semi-normal life.

Surgery was scheduled for that morning since it was currently the middle of the night and the night shift surgeon had already put in a full shift. We would wait for a shift change and more information but, in the meantime, we could get a room and maybe some rest.

Cole and I were admitted to our home away from home, the oncology floor, around 5 AM and greeted by our favorite nurses. The surgery was scheduled for some point during the day. They were unsure of when they would call him for surgery because he was being put on standby which basically meant he was on a waiting list and when the surgeon was finished with a case, he would complete Cole's procedure.

Our assigned surgeon was fairly new to the hospital and no one really knew too much about him. Of course, I asked every single question I could about this mysterious doctor because if he was going to cut my child open, I needed to know his competency in the task.

Around 7 AM, a nurse came into the room and said they were getting Cole ready for surgery, that a Dr. Coppola was opening another operating room and taking Cole's case immediately. I didn't even have much time to call my husband.

Cole and I went down to the pre-op area, my cousin Jess came to meet us, and Josh made it just in time. Jess works in the OR mostly with adults but knew Dr. Coppola's reputation as one of the best pediatric surgeons in the hospital who was meticulous, took his time, and made sure to do everything possible to prevent infection. Upon hearing accolades from several nurses and other doctors on our way to the pre-op area, I immediately knew God placed Dr. Coppola in our lives for a reason.

When I finally met Dr. Coppola moments before my son was going to be under his healing hands, I was immediately struck by his calm, experienced, and intelligent nature. The respect all his nurses and colleagues had for him was evident in the way they assured me that Cole was in good hands and Dr. Coppola was an amazing surgeon. This is one of those events that I can't explain other than saying that God pushed away obstacles and made a way for us to have the best possible scenario.

At that point, everyone, including the surgeon, thought it was a routine appendectomy. Well, nothing with Cole ever seems to be routine. So, we weren't completely surprised when it turned out that his appendix did indeed rupture and was full of infection. I'll remind you that at this point

Cole was still in cancer treatment and had a compromised immune system, so hearing this is nothing short of frightening. But wait. God did something else.

Remember when I mentioned that the ultrasound showed something not quite right with Cole's colon and intestine which triggered the ER doctor to order a CT scan? Well, it was actually Cole's colon that flipped over onto his appendix and created a seal. All the infection and nastiness were under the colon, creating a vacuum seal like situation, so the infection did not spread throughout his body. This, coupled with the last minute open operating room and change of surgeon was truly a miracle.

In the days that followed, as Cole recovered, I got to know our surgeon a little more. He would come in and check on Cole, making sure that everything was going well. This brilliant man who earned his title to the fullest extent insisted I call him Chris. I was raised in an Italian family where we believe title is equal to respect, so I never did, but I was also interested to find out that Dr. Coppola (or Chris) from surgery as he liked to use, was a pediatric surgeon in Iraq where he was stationed while in the military. He performed countless operations on Iraqi children and wrote a book about his experience. I am forever grateful he opened the OR that day and took my son's case.

Going through something as serious as pediatric cancer and its scary, unpredictable treatment side effects put into perspective how even when things seem really dark and down in the pit of despair or the bottom of a roller coaster hill, I truly believe there is someone behind the scenes putting everything into place and moving all obstacles out of the way. Our experiences are proof. Dr. Coppola could have easily been assigned another patient on standby and not Cole. At the time, Cole's case was considered a routine appendectomy. For some reason, everything aligned, and Cole had an experienced and meticulous surgeon to clear out the infection and ensure he was on the road to recovery.

Cole's body also protected him. No one I talked to has ever seen a colon flip and seal away the infection. Again, it was a bad situation that caused a lot of pain, a seven-day hospital stay and tons of anxiety, but looking back on the situation, everything was put in place as if someone in the clouds was moving everything and everyone where they needed to be to protect my child.

The few weeks that followed our discharge from the hospital were nerve-racking to say the least. In order to make sure the EBV wasn't in Cole's lymph nodes, he needed to undergo multiple CT scans and blood tests. The inflammation and infection in his appendix area were assessed and a follow-up CT scan a few weeks later was scheduled. Cole needed to drink a contrast solution which didn't taste like much of anything, but allowed any inflammation to light up like a Christmas tree.

After determining that the EBV was contained to the appendix and since the appendix was removed, we did not need to endure the immunotherapy that would have been necessary if his lymph nodes were compromised. A horrible complication that could have taken my child's life was halted in place and taken care of with expert hands and a few miracles from above.

The nurses, doctors, child life specialist, social worker and everyone else in the hospital were completely aware that Cole reacted to many things and the rare reactions were what plagued my son. Needing to have his appendix removed was one thing, but having the cause be the virus responsible for mono was another weird, full-circle situation.

Cole's pediatrician thought he had mono prior to diagnosis and just tested for leukemia to cover all the bases. Even though it ended up not being mono and was indeed leukemia, the life-threatening reaction that ultimately propelled us to make the decision to end treatment at two years and four months was absolutely due to the mono virus.

No one knows what lies ahead for any of us. In the childhood cancer journey, there is always a possibility of long-term and late onset side effects from the treatment. Though always in the back of my mind, I continually try to push it farther and farther to the back of the room, in the corner, or down the stairs, wherever it fits to allow my mind to heal and my anxiety to decrease. I am aware of the possible side effects, but I am also aware that there was no choice in treatment and the protocol we were given was the best chance of a positive outcome. So, we move forward, "one day at a time", and deal with everything as it comes while advocating for safer treatments in the future.

Cole

Cancer is a pretty awful disease, and the medicine used to treat it is even worse. Even though I was in remission a month after I started treatment, I still needed to get chemo for years to make sure the cancer was gone. Some of the side effects of the chemo were bad. It wasn't bad enough that the cancer made me sick, but the chemo made me even sicker at some points.

The steroids were pretty bad too, and they weren't even chemotherapy. I needed to take them about once a month for around a week each time. The first part of treatment, the steroid I took made me very hungry, angry, itchy, and I couldn't sleep. I didn't like the way it made me feel and I couldn't relax the entire time I took them. It seemed like I was hungry all the time and I craved certain snacks like chips and pretzels, but I got heartburn almost every day and my stomach was upset easily. After I told my doctors about the heartburn, I started taking another medicine to help with that and even something to coat my throat and stomach to help with my stomachache. They also made my face very puffy.

Towards the end of the main part of treatment I developed diabetes because of all the steroids and a certain type of chemo that was given at the same time as the steroids. My mom had to inject me with insulin up to three times a day depending on what my sugar was. I didn't really get upset or care much. It was just another little poke, but I did not like getting my sugar checked. The needles made my fingers very sore.

I realize that this was a pretty difficult time of treatment. A lot of reactions occurred around the same time, I was hospitalized frequently and spent many nights in the emergency department. I knew, in the back of my mind, that I was nearing the end of the hardest part of treatment but it was still very hard. I didn't know what to expect during maintenance, but my doctors and nurses kept telling me that it was going to get easier really soon. I kept pushing through and reminded myself that I was almost there.

During the last two phases of frontline treatment, my body was extremely tired from the months of treatment I endured. Also, my counts took a lot longer to recover. The doctors said it was because my bone marrow was bombarded with chemo and the closer we got to maintenance, the harder it was for the marrow (and the counts) to return close to normal due to the repeated doses. This is what they wanted and I just needed to remember maintenance was right around the corner.

In November of 2020, ten long months after diagnosis, I finally reached the phase I had been looking forward to since starting treatment. During maintenance, there were a lot of changes for the better. First, the steroid I was on now (prednisone) didn't cause as many side effects and I could hardly tell the difference in myself when I was on steroid week. This also meant that my blood sugar didn't rise and I didn't need to be on insulin any longer. I was very happy that my sugar was stable and insulin, blood sugar checks, and being thirsty all the time stopped.

Also, I wasn't as hungry all the time and was able to focus on eating better and getting healthy. I lost all the weight I put on during the last ten months and was feeling a lot better. I definitely slept better and wasn't up all night anymore like with the previous steroid. Even though I noticed my mood did change slightly with this medicine, I didn't get nearly as angry as I used to be with the other steroid.

I was glad the prednisone was easier to handle because I needed to be on this medication once a month for the next three years. I don't want to think how different my life would have been if there wasn't a different steroid option and I needed to continue with the dexamethasone for over three more years.

I tolerated most medications well. However, there were a few medicines that made me really nauseous. The methotrexate I needed towards the end of the main treatment caused me to be hospitalized. I was so nauseous that I couldn't keep anything down (including water). I needed to go to the hospital for fluids because I was so dehydrated. I also developed sores all over my body, in my mouth and all the way down my throat into my stomach. My skin looked like it was burned and felt like the worst sunburn imaginable. I couldn't walk or even move without pain. I couldn't even have clothes touch my skin. Nothing helped the pain, not even morphine. I was on a few different medicines to help clear up the sores and it took a couple of weeks 'til I was comfortable again.

The methotrexate reaction, along with my allergic reaction to PEG-asparaginase, were the two worst experiences during frontline treatment. The PEG reaction was super scary and I don't remember too much about it, but I remember throwing up and then getting the EPIPEN® injection in my leg. I was afraid I would react to this chemo from the very beginning because I knew it was a possibility, and my doctors and nurses asked me to let them know if anything felt off each time they started the chemo. I was almost happy when I reacted the last time because I knew I didn't need to get that chemo ever again. Well, I was relieved, at least until the Erwinase® shots began. They were the most painful experience I had during treatment.

Most of the other chemotherapy just made me very tired and made my counts low which meant I couldn't really go anywhere and had to be really careful not to get sick. Most of the reactions and sickness ended with the aggressive chemo and maintenance was definitely much easier. I remained out of the hospital, my counts returned to above 1,000 and I was almost back to normal until May of 2022.

I didn't even realize my last side effect was due to chemotherapy and my suppressed immune system. Let me describe what happened, step-by-step, in May 2022 which led to a long hospital stay and ultimately an early end of treatment celebration. In the spring of 2022, I was throwing for our track and field team. I was finally starting to feel more like myself and when my doctors allowed me to participate in track, I jumped on the opportunity. I mentioned before how much I love sports and I was really missing the ability to participate. I knew my body wasn't ready for running, so I settled on throwing and participated in all events available like javelin, shot put, and discus. Towards the end of the season, I developed really bad pain in my side and I thought I pulled a muscle due to all the throwing I was doing the last couple months.

However, the pain didn't go away. It kept getting worse. Actually, the day I went to the hospital the pain was so bad that I couldn't walk or even stand without holding my side to try to support myself and lessen the stabbing pain. At this point, I also developed a fever, so I knew we needed to go to the hospital. I'm pretty sure pulled muscles don't give you a fever so I knew it was something more serious.

After my mom took my temperature and realized it was almost 103 degrees, she took me to the emergency room. I remember it was pretty late at night when we got there and all I wanted to do was sleep. The hospital is not a very comfortable place to sleep, so I really didn't get any rest. I was taken for a few tests like an ultrasound, bloodwork and a CT scan so the doctors could see what was happening. The ultrasound tech came right into my ER room and did her scan. She couldn't really see my appendix which is what the doctor thought was responsible for my pain and fever. So, a CT scan was ordered where they finally found out I had an appendicitis and I needed to have my appendix removed. I was really upset. I was finally getting back to normal, and I had less than a year left in treatment. I was going to need surgery and be in the hospital once again. I was really afraid of starting over again and being in the hospital yet again.

Everything happened really quickly and I was taken into surgery the following morning. My surgeon was amazing and was able to take out my appendix (which ruptured by the way) and only give me a small scar through my belly button. I was pretty nervous about getting an infection and having to be in the hospital even longer, but all the nurses and my oncologist told me my surgeon was very careful and took extra care to make sure he got everything. This made me feel better, knowing I had one of the best surgeons in the hospital.

I remember everyone being so surprised at how bad my appendix was ruptured and that I wasn't in more pain. I still have the picture my surgeon gave me of my stomach when he opened it and saw what was underneath. I thought it was cool that he had a machine to take pictures while doing the surgery.

My recovery from surgery was the most difficult time of treatment. The first day or so after surgery was ok, but as the medication and anesthesia wore off, the extreme pain started. I was unable to move and all the medication I was given didn't help to ease the pain. My nurses wanted me to get up and walk, so the day after surgery I did. I was able to walk around the hospital floor and felt ok. However, something happened the following day, and the pain was so bad I could barely get out of bed. I became so nauseous and I was terrified to throw up because my stomach was just cut open and I couldn't imagine the amount of pain vomiting would cause.

The third or fourth day after surgery is when I starting vomiting. I couldn't eat and I was so nauseous. There wasn't anything that helped. The doctors tried a patch behind my ear and Zofran® but nothing took it away. My nurse later told me due to the surgery and the pain medication my intestines slowed down and made me really nauseous. This lasted a couple of days and finally stopped. When the nausea went away I was able to get up and walk a little at a time and finally eat. I lost a lot of weight before and after my surgery which took a long time to gain.

Two days before I was discharged from the hospital, my oncologist Dr. Miller, came into my room and told us that my appendix tested positive for EBV. I wasn't sure what that meant, but it did make me pretty nervous. At that point, I just wanted to feel better and stop having these reactions and hospital stays. My doctor and my parents explained everything to me in a way that I understood.

I was exposed to the virus responsible for mono, Epstein–Barr virus. In a person with a normal immune system, they probably wouldn't even notice. It may cause a sore throat or cold. However, since my immune system was suppressed by chemo when I was exposed, the virus confused my lymphocytes which are the cells in your blood that fight infections. Instead of the lymphocytes attacking the virus they started dividing like crazy and attacked my appendix.

When I got out of the hospital, I needed some CT scans and blood tests to make sure the EBV didn't spread throughout my body and just stayed in my appendix which was now gone. The doctors had a plan if the EBV was in my body but they assured me we would figure everything out and we would talk about what we needed to do after the tests were complete.

Since this reaction to EBV was very rare and my doctors only treated transplant recipients with this particular reaction, not cancer patients, they talked to doctors from a larger hospital, CHOP. This hospital had a doctor that specialized in this type of reaction. From what my doctor told me, the doctor at the other hospital explained that they recently started a new protocol for boys with my type of cancer.

At my hospital, girls get two years of maintenance and boys get three years of maintenance. Since CHOP is the hospital doing the research, they were able to move both boys and girls to two years of maintenance earlier than some other hospitals. The doctors felt it was necessary to do this for me to prevent any more reactions in the future. The doctors felt it was safer to stop my treatment than wait for anymore side effects to occur, so I was able to end treatment in October instead of May. I was so relieved to be done with the chemotherapy and able to get back to my normal life after three long years.

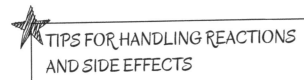

TIPS FOR HANDLING REACTIONS AND SIDE EFFECTS

Parents/Caregivers
Get all the information necessary to be prepared for what may happen.

Ask lots and lots of questions, about everything.

You cannot advocate for your child if you don't ask and push when something isn't right.

Stay calm. Yeah right! How about appear like you are calm. If you are upset, your child will be upset so acting as level-headed as possible in front of them when they are experiencing something unpleasant can help the fight.

Supporters
Cancer is awful, sticky, messy, and downright evil. So, it's understandable that to kill cancer, chemo has to be pretty awful too.

Give support when needed.

You don't need to understand, sometimes just listening helps.

Check in once in a while if possible, and give the family what they need to refuel for the rest of the journey.

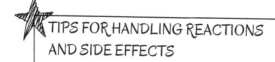

TIPS FOR HANDLING REACTIONS AND SIDE EFFECTS

<u>Side Effects We Experienced & What Helped Us</u>

Mucositis - Magic Mouth Wash, prescribed by the doctors to numb the throat and create a coating to help ease swallowing.

Helios - we didn't hear about this product until afterwards, but I've heard good things. Make sure to consult your team first. I believe they also send a free box to cancer patients.

Nausea – Zofran which is prescribed by the doctor and one of the only things that worked for nausea.

Queasy Pops – can be purchased online or in many stores.

Ginger chews

Nausea bands

Scopalmine patch - prescribed by the doctor for extreme nausea after appendicitis.

Benadryl - yes, it's an allergy medication but also used to combat nausea.

Heartburn - PEPCID® - prescribed by a doctor to help with heartburn from steroids.

Caution against using TUMS- we were told to avoid them

Itchiness - Cortizone cream for rashes and extreme itchiness (prescribed by our team).

Ice- if a spot became really itchy sometimes ice would help.

Skin reactions - Creams prescribed by our team

Switching bandages - Avoiding adhesives

Switching port dressing to IV 3000

Neutropenia Protocols - Vary from hospital to hospital. Typically, there is a minimum temperature like 100.5 and then you take it again an hour later. If it's the same or higher, the team should be called. However, if the temperature is above a certain degree (ours was around 101.7), you call immediately. No need to wait and recheck.

Sanitize! - I used to joke that I had a holster of Lysol spray and a wipe dispenser. Everything should be wiped frequently when counts are low. Pay special attention to light switches, handles, and doorknobs, phone and video game controllers (anything that is touched regularly).

Avoid sick people.

Wear masks in public.

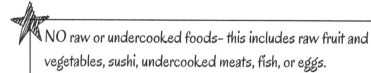

NO raw or undercooked foods- this includes raw fruit and vegetables, sushi, undercooked meats, fish, or eggs.

No fresh flowers in the house – they can carry germs and contaminants that can be harmful to an immunocompromised person.

Disclaimer - We are not medical professionals. Be sure to consult your team before implementing any of these strategies. They may also have additional tips and tricks. We are simply sharing our unique story and what we did that helped us.

CHAPTER 6

Beauty in the Broken
Beautiful Things During Difficult Times

There is beauty in the broken. Sometimes the most beautiful things happen in the ugliest and darkest of places.

Laura

Even though this road is difficult and often treacherous, there are beautifully scenic areas of the journey. I'm immediately faced with an image of the most beautiful, blue tinted clear ocean waters with the whitest and smoothest sand I've ever seen. The sky is also blue, without even the smallest hint of haziness. In fact, the sky is so clear it's almost translucent. As I stand next to my car which is pulled over in a safe alcove, I look over the edge of the cliff at the road below that I took to get to this location. There are so many twists and turns and downright scary areas of this one lane road with two lane traffic that I almost can't believe I made it to this beautiful point in the journey.

While I am now safe and sound admiring a beautiful view, I realize that one wrong step and I can tumble down the cliff into the perils below. The safety I experience now may not last and in order to continue on the journey to the end, I must get back on the dangerous road and continue driving and leading my family through this experience.

So many things have occurred in the last three years that took my car entirely too close to the edge of the road or steered it face-to-face with oncoming traffic. Whatever the treacherous experience may have been, it was downright terrifying and dangerous. Each time we were placed in a precarious position, everything worked out perfectly and we were able to exit the vehicle safely and observe the beauty in the brokenness. There is no one other than God who can orchestrate such a beautiful symphony of circumstances at exactly the right time. One of the main reasons I was able to get through the dark days is my faith and signs from above that let me know that God was walking before our family and making a way for us through this cancer journey.

One thing that helps strengthen my faith is to know that God and Jesus do not talk to us by using actual words. Language is how humans communicate with each other. God uses signs to show us we are seen and loved. The signs we were given during our journey showed up at the perfect time and propelled us through the broken pieces and helped us to keep going. The signs we experienced were so beautiful and breathtaking that we are grateful God pulled us to safety so we could admire the beauty in front of us.

I fully realize that many people have different beliefs and I am not using this book to sway you one way or another. I am, however, sharing our story and how I coped with the trauma and heartbreaking events of the past three years. This chapter of our story takes some of the signs and angels sent to us and explains exactly how they picked us up and set us back on our feet to continue on the next leg of the arduous journey.

I already shared two beautiful stories regarding two angels I met before our cancer life who showed up at the exact time I needed them. My classmate and a coworker during my internship at the middle school were there for me in the hospital during Cole's diagnosis and initial hospital stay. In addition to these two individuals, a church friend whose son was also one of our nurses, and countless other friends who worked at the hospital, all showed concern for our family.

I want to share with you a few other experiences we had along our journey which significantly impacted our lives and continue to do so. In the previous chapter regarding side effects, I talked about a few side effects Cole experienced, but I wanted to save the PEG-asparaginase reaction for this chapter because even though it was a dark and scary time it correlates with one of the most beautiful experiences in our journey.

PEG-asparaginase was the primary chemotherapy drug used during very strategic parts of Cole's treatment to kill cancer cells by starving them at a precise time and in a precise way. This potent chemical was made using E-coli bacteria. Yep, the E-coli that can make a person super sick or even kill them. This is the type of poison we are talking about, and it was intentionally injected into my son's port to kill the cancer. Known to cause problems and often anaphylactic reactions, nurses and medical professionals are armed with a kit containing various things like an EPIPEN® and other medications to reverse this drug and save the patient's life in the event of an adverse reaction while receiving the infusion.

Since many patients react to this particular drug, there is an alternate medication. At the time of Cole's treatment, there was only one alternate and it was Erwinase®. Due to the volatile nature of the drug, since the process to create Erwinase® used a plant-based bacteria Erwinia Chrysanthemi, equally as dangerous as E-Coli, manufacturing this poison needed to be extremely precise. Since the ingredients of this chemo can be very dangerous, the process takes about nine months for one batch. If even the slightest error is made, the batch is discarded and months of work is wasted.

The long process, coupled with the fact that many kids were reacting to PEG-asparaginase, and only one company was producing the backup drug, landed the poison on the National Drug Shortage List. Great. Not only did my child just go through a harrowing experience that threatened his life, now the poison that was going to kill the cancer, and very important to his treatment plan, was unavailable. There wasn't a favorable possible outcome without this drug. If this wasn't a dangerous cliff adjacent road with little room for safety, I'm not sure what situation qualifies as dangerous.

Even though I was told of this possibility when starting the PEG, as it was called, I naively thought we wouldn't be affected by the shortage. Wow, was I wrong. Cole was scheduled to receive around 10 rounds of this drug. He received four rounds, reacting during the fourth administration of the drug. Since the backup poison was on the shortage list, hospital policy was to re-challenge patients who reacted to a certain degree.

So, Cole was admitted into the PICU for the day and watched under the close eye of one of our favorite nurses, Gary. The drug was administered at half speed, meaning that if it normally took an hour, this time it would take two. Cole also received Benadryl and steroids before the IV infusion started, a combination aimed to thwart any type of adverse event.

While Gary and I chatted like long lost friends, Cole slept through the treatment due to the sleepy effect from Benadryl. He woke as we were ready to leave with red and puffy eyes and a tingling face. One of our oncologists was called into the room and instructed a second dose of Benadryl could be given. So, Gary gave Cole the medicine and we were on our way home.

Fast forward one week, Cole developed a fever, body aches and was shaking uncontrollably with the chills. Per protocol, I called the oncologist immediately and we were on our way to the ER a few minutes later. To put this into perspective, it was the end of March 2020 when COVID-19 was new and extremely scary.

So, having to go to the hospital with a fever in that time was terrifying beyond the normal scary cancer stuff. The oncologist on call happened to be the same doctor that saw us a week prior during the re-challenge in the PICU. She called the ER and alerted them that we would be coming. Since Cole did have a fever, we didn't have to wait in the waiting room which would have possibly exposed us to some scary germs and illnesses.

When we arrived at the hospital, there was a tent outside the ER where our temperatures were checked and written on wristbands. Since Cole had a fever (I believe it was around 102), he was transported to the ER door in a golf cart, and we were immediately taken to a vacuum sealed room and locked away from others.

The nurse arrived sometime later with a jet pack type device and sterile suit to protect her from us in case Cole was positive for COVID-19. The possibility of this was low and all signs pointed to a neutropenic fever which is a fever brought on by low blood counts. Still, we needed a negative test before all was deemed safe. It took 24 hours of a sealed PICU room, many jet pack nurses, and minimal human contact before our negative result and a transfer to a normal hospital room upstairs.

What I failed to mention is that Cole's blood pressure bottomed out and was extremely low. He needed medication to bring it up, which was the reason we were in PICU from the start, coupled with the fact that they had the sealed rooms we needed until our results came back and our hematology/oncology floor did not.

Original thoughts from the PICU doctor were sepsis due to the extremely low blood pressure. But, guess what? PEG can cause this exact type of drop in blood pressure, and he already reacted twice to this medication. Being that he received the dose a week prior, and the medication stays in the system two weeks AND no sepsis ever showed on his blood cultures. Ding, ding, ding, PEG reaction number three.

It was still never confirmed, and all inquiries made to the doctor regarding a PEG reaction were dismissed because we couldn't prove it 100% and this drug was important. Cole received the next dose of poison in clinic since the re-challenge was deemed successful and the hospital stay was attributed to some other mystical occurrence. I was naïve and scared and didn't know what to do, so I went along with professional advice and kept moving forward in treatment because the alternative was terrifying with the backup drug unavailable.

About 20 minutes into a two-hour infusion with pre-meds as a precaution, Cole reacted. He began vomiting and was extremely weak. This part may be hard to read because it was a nightmare to experience.

Cole started to yell out "help me, help me Mom" over and over as his arms were flailing. He was grabbing onto me as he began to fall backwards onto the treatment table. His eyes rolled in the back of his head and he looked like he was fainting. In the blink of an eye, we were surrounded by nurses and doctors moving furiously around the room as I held my son's hand. I heard the doctors give the nurses clear instructions and the medication was stopped immediately. Cole's blood pressure was also taken. It was extremely low and getting lower. I heard Denise ask our doctor if she should give Cole an injection. He nodded yes and our angel nurse Denise took control and grabbed the EPIPEN®, plunging it into Cole's thigh.

A few minutes after the injection, his pressure began to rise and he was stable. I'll never forget Dr Yohannes telling me that he was going to make it. I never ever even considered that my child could have died in that clinic because of this medication. I am still in denial and push it away because it's unimaginable. I am equally puzzled by the circumstances surrounding the reaction.

Due to a drug shortage in the United States where we are supposed to have access to life-saving medication, my son was exposed to an allergen three separate times after his first reaction. If the back-up medication was available and things were simple, one reaction should be all it takes to qualify a child to receive an alternate life-saving medication.

Finally, this reaction was enough to qualify Cole as allergic and no longer subject to this poison. I honestly still can't believe everything Cole needed to go through due to this drug shortage. All of these events occurred before he was put on Erwinase® to ensure he could get all of the chemo he needed in case we couldn't locate Erwinase®. Now that Cole was officially deemed allergic to PEG-asparaginase, we were officially on the hunt for Erwinase®.

The first dose was able to be purchased without much trouble, but I was told that the shortage was going to increase, and it was going to become nearly impossible to find. I had a couple of weeks until it was needed. So, I began asking the staff what I could do and how we were going to find this medication. Their hands were tied. They couldn't go on the search because they were bound to rules and regulations, however, I was not. I was a mom of a very sick child who was not going to take no for an answer. I began calling everyone I could think of: my political representatives, people at other hospitals and the pharmaceutical company responsible for the medication.

I was connected to a lovely woman at the pharmaceutical company who kept me informed of when the batches would be released in hopes that I could alert our pediatric oncology pharmacist at our small hospital and the clinic could get their hands on the vials we needed.

At one point, the vials were unattainable, and I did not know what to do.

By the grace of God, the pharmaceutical company connected us to Laura Bray. Laura went through the same shortage a few months prior with her daughter Abby. She worked so hard to get the medicine Abby needed and was so moved by the experience that she started her own nonprofit organization to help other families experiencing a drug shortage. *Angels for Change* was born from a mother's love and determination to do anything necessary to help her daughter obtain her life-saving medication.

I sent *Angels for Change* an email explaining our situation and was immediately contacted via telephone by Laura herself. We must have talked for over an hour regarding our story and her story and the situation we were currently experiencing with the drug shortage.

This was the first of many phone calls and the beginning of a friendship that continues today. At one point in the conversation, Laura asked if she could pray with me. I immediately felt at ease and a temporary peace come over me with a feeling that we were going to find the medication we needed for Cole. Laura got to work immediately, contacting the pharmaceutical company, the medication distributor, several hospitals, the FDA and every other connection she made over the last nine months in the attempt to find any vials that were available for the hospital to purchase.

The task I asked of Laura was profound. Cole needed over 100 vials of a medication that was nowhere to be found. It was essential to his treatment, and I don't even dare to think of what would have happened had she not been successful in her search.

We remained in constant contact over the next five cycles of the medication. One of my friends from high school happened to be in charge of the pediatric pharmacy department at our hospital. I reached out immediately to connect her to Laura. Since I was going through a life-threatening situation and extremely close to everything that was happening, I tried to reach out to everyone I knew, not worrying about the details or effects.

Due to protocol and procedure, my friend was hesitant to work with Laura until speaking with her and realizing the work Laura was able to accomplish by following proper procedures, building connections, and always utilizing the proper avenues.

From the initial contact on, my friend worked directly with Laura, and they were able to go through the proper channels to find the medicine. I am forever grateful to everyone who worked so hard to help us. There are so many details, unexplained events, and connections I've had work together to create a positive outcome many times during our journey, and this is one that definitively sticks out.

Receiving the vials of chemo was only part of the battle. Since the medication is extremely potent and painful to receive, Cole was faced with two difficult challenges. The painful injections, which were the preferred way of administering the medicine, and the awful side effects including nausea and diabetes.

To further explain our ordeal, I need to describe what receiving this medication was like for Cole. The PEG was able to be given via IV, but with the Erwinase®, the suggested method of administration is IM injection, which is an inter muscular injection as opposed to a regular cutaneous (skin) injection like the flu shot.

The IM shot is administered into a muscle rather than the skin for better absorption into the bloodstream and increased effectiveness of the medication. Because of Cole's size (at the time he was 14 and 15 years old and well over 150 pounds), Cole needed two injections each time. The course of the medication was Monday, Wednesday, and Friday for two weeks. In case I've lost you already, for each course of this medication, Cole needed 12 injections. He had three courses to go, so we began the countdown at 36 shots.

One of our nurses, Barbie, described these shots as the least favorite part of her job. The medication burned going in, like a "make a grown man cry" burn. Ice and numbing medication didn't touch the inferno coursing through my child's legs. He never cried, but he made the worst face and squeezed the life out my hand. I wished there was another way, something else that could be done, but I am eternally grateful that we were able to obtain this vicious monster to complete his treatment plan.

Everyone worked together to make this experience less painful for Cole including picking out the most ridiculous BAND-AIDs® to get a smile from my child. Our favorite depicted a yellow minion with an octopus stuck to its face with the words "this sucks" above the cartoon. Everyone laughed and thought they were absolutely the perfect depiction of the process. His child life specialist at the time, Ashley, even got Cole a balloon that said "You did it", the nurses made him a minion themed sign and they all signed it in awe of Cole's accomplishment and completion of 36 injections marking the end of frontline treatment and a new phase of the journey: maintenance.

The beauty in this difficult experience is the people I've connected with and brought together for a specific purpose. I am extremely proud to call many of them friends. They are amazing individuals.

Laura Bray used to say frequently during our initial conversations that she is just a mom. No, she is not just anything. Yes, she is a mom, but she is also a business woman with the specific knowledge and skills who made the choice to do something about a significant problem affecting her daughter. She continued to make a choice to use that knowledge and connections to help others. Because of her choice, my son received the medication he needed, and he was not the only one she helped.

The Erwinase® shortage is currently resolved due to the pressure Laura put on many companies and organizations. The decision was made to develop another alternate drug which was in the trial stage at the time of our search. The trials were completed, and the product launched in perfect timing. We were able to help one patient get on the trial at our hospital and Laura has helped countless others receive this medicine on time and save them from experiencing the awful re-challenge and reaction ordeal Cole had to go through. Now, patients who react to PEG shouldn't need to be put through re-challenges, exposing them to potentially life-threatening reactions. Nor should they have to walk on eggshells waiting for a batch of medication very hard to come by in the hopes that their hospital was able to secure the amount needed. RYLAZE® is made using a process much faster than nine months, solving the issue of low supply/high demand.

The number of amazing things *Angels for Change* has accomplished warms my heart. During one of the most difficult parts of Cole's treatment journey and probably one of the lowest points for me, I found an angel who helped us and picked up the phone when I was panicking. Through her harrowing personal experience with her daughter, she made a choice to use that pain and brokenness to help others.

Though my heart and soul were broken at many points throughout our treatment journey, this was one experience when I can say it was mended with the friendship and bond of another mother willing to advocate for other pediatric cancer patients. I will always advocate for other families going through this horrible experience because I will always remember that I was that mom, broken, alone, and in despair. Another mom picked me up and dusted me off so I will always repay the kindness.

Another story of beauty in the broken lies at the hospital where we were treated. I mentioned previously in the book that my cousin, Jess, works at the hospital in the OR. At the time, her department was part of Interventional Radiology (IR), and is the department usually responsible for placing ports in patients. The group of people she worked with are extremely close and supportive. There are several amazing things that happened through Jessie and her co-workers. The first act of kindness happened shortly after Cole's diagnosis. Maggie, one of Jessie's co-workers approached her and asked if it was okay if she gave us a check. Jess immediately called and explained the situation before asking me if it would be ok.

You see, Maggie's son just turned two years old and the previous year when he turned one they had everyone contribute to a cause close to the family's heart in lieu of gifts. It turns out they did the same thing this year and raised money again instead of accepting gifts. Maggie wanted to donate the money to us. We were the family she and her husband chose to be the recipient of the donations this year. I was stunned. I never met Maggie, but did hear about her often through Jess since they worked very close together. We, of course, accepted and thanked her profusely.
The compassion this amazing family showed to our family when we were at rock bottom is amazing and will never be forgotten. So, when Cole rang the bell on Oct 3, 2022, Jess and Maggie were there to witness the ceremony. I gave her a huge hug and thanked her again for her kindness at the beginning of our journey. I was so glad she was able to be there for such a monumental accomplishment; the end of chemo.

Countless other coworkers, nurses, doctors and surgeons that work with Jess looked out for us during our journey. Not only did they look out for Cole and our entire family, but they eased Jessie's mind and supported her as she was trying to support us and help us navigate such a trying time. Cole is Jessie's god-son and he is the first grandchild on my side of the family. Our family is extremely close and supportive, through good and bad. So, I knew Jess would stop at nothing to help us and be there even if she was struggling herself. I am grateful to her colleagues for not only looking out for us but for supporting Jessie when I was too broken to support myself.

Many other beautiful acts of kindness reached our family at exactly the right moment. Another person I worked with at the middle school, a gifted school counselor dropped off pediatric cancer themed nail wraps and jewelry when we were in the throes of the Erwinase® crisis. A parent of one of Cole's friends put a gift card in the mail for one of our favorite restaurants. We received it when we got home from a particularly difficult hospital admission. Many other people sent cards, prayers, well-wishes and gift packages which always seemed to come during the storm and helped us see the light in the darkness.

Once again, I cannot explain any of these beautiful events that pulled us from our brokenness but I know they happened and I know who is responsible for showing us the signs we needed at that particular moment. Right when it seemed like we couldn't go any further or swim in the struggle any longer, a life-line was thrown and we held on filling ourselves with as much strength as possible to keep going.

Cole

After the shock of my diagnosis wore off, I knew I needed to summon all my strength to get through this long battle. Cancer, and everything that comes with it, is the hardest thing I've ever gone through in my life. Since it is such an awful disease, sometimes it's hard to think about the good things that happened during that time, but it's important to remember all the amazing things and people who helped get me through a trying time and hard battle.

There are a few things that happened during treatment that helped push me to keep going. The doctors, nurses, and child life specialists who helped me during treatment are a big part of my journey and I couldn't have done it without them. They tried everything to help and make me feel comfortable. My nurses were amazing and always tried to make me laugh and smile even by doing something small like giving me snacks or picking out funny bandages. Some days it was the little things that helped the most, especially when we were at the hospital all day.

Our clinic is pretty small, so I had the same three nurses throughout my entire treatment. Some left for other jobs, but there were always three nurses in the clinic. Barbie is one of those amazing nurses and she and Meg were the only two that were there from day one. Barbie has been in that clinic for over 40 years and is one of the nicest people I've ever met. She is from the town where I lived when I was younger and where most of my family still lives. She is a tiny lady with a big personality, and you can hear her all the way down the hall. I felt a little calmer when I heard her call my name from the hallway before I could see her. She always seemed to make the hard days easier and she was very good at her job. I never had to worry when Barbie accessed my port because she did it so well. With my second port, I had a great experience so it didn't really bother me to get accessed. The first port, however, was a different story. It never really healed right and sometimes it was more difficult to access. Barbie always got it even though it wasn't easy for her some days.

All my nurses did a great job at explaining everything they were doing in a way that I could understand. They took as much time as needed to make sure I was comfortable. Since we spent so much time at the hospital, we got to know the doctors and nurses very well and they always asked questions about what was going on in my life outside of treatment which showed that they really cared about me and wanted to get to know me well.

My child life specialist was another person who really helped me by distracting me and making sure I wasn't too bored. She wasn't in the clinic for the first part of my treatment, but she was in pediatric sedation and always talked to me about video games and made sure to give me a funny hairstyle that I could laugh at when I woke up after anesthesia. When she came to clinic, she made me do crafts with her, talked about our favorite video games and shows, and tried to distract me as much as possible.

Her sister also went through a leukemia diagnosis when she was younger, so I felt like Rose knew exactly what it was like for me to experience this treatment. I'm glad she told me about her sister, and I realize that is why she decided to become a child life specialist. She is very good at her job, and I appreciated all the attention she gave me. She actually came to my last track meet of the season to see me throw.

When I was in the clinic a few days before the meet, she asked where it was and what time and I thought she was joking when she said she would be there. Nope. She definitely came and cheered me on. When she showed up and stood in the field with my mom, I smiled because I couldn't believe she would take the time, outside of work, to come and watch me throw. At that moment, I knew my whole team was super special and felt supported and cared for in a way I could never imagine.

Without my amazing team, I wouldn't be where I am today. So many people worked together during my treatment, and I needed to be seen by many different areas in the hospital. Everyone was helpful and kind. My mom also tried everything she could to make the experience easier. Being in the hospital almost everyday is not fun for anyone. So, I really appreciate everything my family, friends, and medical team did to make each day a little brighter.

One really nerve-wracking part of treatment was when I reacted to PEG and then found out we couldn't find the chemo I needed for the remainder of my treatment. Since I already started this medication, I didn't qualify for a clinical trial of a new, similar medicine to PEG, so I was really nervous that they wouldn't be able to find all the medicine I needed.

After three courses of the medicine, our hospital couldn't find anymore. My mom called everyone she could think of, including the pharmaceutical company that made the medicine, and was connected to a foundation whose purpose was to find life-saving medicine on the drug shortage list when hospitals had a hard time finding it.

Laura Bray and *Angels for Change* found all the chemo for me. I was very grateful because I knew I needed the chemo to get better even though getting the shots was the most painful experience of my treatment. I knew I had to push through the pain of the shots and get to the other side. During a scary point in treatment, when I didn't know if I was going to have the medicine I needed, and what it would mean if they couldn't find it, everything aligned and all the medicine was found.

My friends also helped me a lot through my journey. I knew I could lean on them if I needed someone, and they would always be there for me. Even though they didn't understand what I was going through, they still listened and helped in any way they could. It really helped me to play video games with them because most of my treatment was during COVID and even afterwards, when my counts were low, I couldn't really be around many people. Connecting to my friends online via video games helped me to block everything out and act like a normal teenager by escaping through the game.

Another thing that really helped was an organization called 18 Loop who gave me a Quest VR system. The system had calming apps that I could use before a stressful appointment, and I could even add my own games. I still have the system and it's really neat to use. My entire family loves it and I'm grateful to the organization for providing it to me during a rough point in treatment. It really allowed me to escape and forget, if only for a few moments.

Other people that helped me along the way were one of my favorite teachers who came to my house to teach me that first year I was diagnosed. She actually had breast cancer a few years before I was diagnosed, so she did know what I was going through and helped me out a lot. Her encouragement really helped in the first few months of treatment. I felt inspired and got the strength and courage to fight because she did it, and she was doing well now.

She showed me it's possible and I needed to push through the hard days and it would get better. I'll never forget when she showed me a picture of herself with no hair. It was pretty early on in my treatment and I was very nervous to lose my hair. By her showing me how she looked without any hair, it made the possibility of losing my hair not seem as terrifying. She even put together gift baskets for my entire family when I was diagnosed to show us the school supported me.

My class also gave me a mini Jenga® game and each person signed a piece with a message for me. I still pull that game out and read all the pieces and messages each person wrote to me. It helps me when I have a bad day to see how far I have come from the early days of diagnosis. The cards, gifts, signs, stickers, and messages all helped and were a bright spot in my dark journey.

Another thing that helped were the organizations that my mom found to support me. *Project Outrun* was one of them and they gave me the opportunity to design my very own pair of Nike sneakers. I love basketball sneakers and collect different pairs of Nikes so when my mom asked if I wanted to design my own, I was excited. I was in a pretty hard part of treatment at the time, so getting the chance to make something custom like Nike sneakers gave me something to look forward to. I was able to pick the color, style and everything and then it was delivered to me. They also sent me a medal, a T-shirt, and some other things.

There were a couple of other organizations that sent me sports gear and fan gear like T-shirts, sweatshirts, and jerseys of my favorite teams. Though getting these things did not take away all the bad, it made me smile and made it easier to keep going forward. Knowing that others were supporting me and were encouraging me helped me during the worst times.

I don't like to be the center of attention and usually don't ask for things and my mom knew this, so she, along with my child life specialist and social worker and other people close to me, organized everything and surprised me a couple of times.

If you are going through a hard part in treatment, just know that everyone is rooting for you. Take it "one day at a time" and get through the hard day. Talk to your family and friends and let them help support and cheer you on. Sometimes you can't do it all alone. You need an army supporting you and doing amazing things to help you along the way so you can climb the mountain and get to the other side, which is the end of treatment.

WORDS OF ENCOURAGEMENT FOR MOMENTS IN THE BROKEN

Here are some quotes and verses that inspired us during the journey, and we hope that they inspire you as well:

"So do not fear, for I am with you; do not be dismayed, for I am your God. I will strengthen you and help you; I will uphold you with my righteous right hand. " - Isaiah 41:10

"When it rains, look for rainbows. When it's dark, look for stars." – Oscar Wilde

"But those who hope in the Lord will renew their strength. They will soar on wings like eagles; they will run and not grow weary, they will walk and not be faint." - Isaiah 40:31

"Broken crayons still color."

"Even though I walk through the darkest valley, I will fear no evil, for you are with me; your rod and your staff, they comfort me." - Psalm 23:4

"Believe you can and you're halfway there." - Theodore Roosevelt

Take everything One Day at a Time and when that's not possible, take it one hour at a time or one moment at a time. Live in the present.

CHAPTER 7

*Relationships: Cancer Isn't Contagious
But People Act That Way*

In our experience, only those who have been in the pit of despair and experienced a similar trauma can stay and offer support in the worst moments instead of only being there for the best.

Laura

We are an extremely lucky family because we have a supportive (to the point of being way over the top) extended family. Our family is at every one of the boys' sporting events, school functions, and birthday parties. They contribute to every fundraiser and put every picture and project our boys make on the refrigerator. So, our family relationships pretty much stayed the same during and after treatment.

They were there every step of the way, cheering us on, calling with concern when we were admitted, offering thousands and thousands of prayers, bringing food and care baskets, and even running coffee up to our hospital room during their work breaks (thanks Jess).

During Cole's initial hospitalization, I was brought to tears when his two very good friends put on hospital gowns and masks to visit with Cole in the PICU. I can still see the smile on Cole's face when his friends entered his hospital room. They talked, drank soda, and played video games on Cole's PlayStation® the nurses helped us sneak in. Even though his friends were upset to know that Cole had cancer, they showed up and made Cole feel like everything was normal, even if only for a few hours. I can't imagine what was running through these 14-year old's minds, but I am eternally grateful for their care and concern.

Though we had family support, helpful hospital staff, caring friends and the community, I still felt alone at certain points during treatment. As I look back, it was the hardest of times that I felt the most alone. When I thought I couldn't take anymore, I received a call or text from a friend offering their support out of the blue not even knowing was going on at the moment. I felt like I was throwing my dart-like, poignant words right at their hearts when I divulged what we were experiencing. Friends I was very close with before Cole's diagnosis, my fellow warrior moms, Momcology® moms, and my family did not even flinch as these words pierced their heart. They simply removed the darts, asked what I needed, and supported in any way possible.

Somedays I just needed someone else to hear the things we were experiencing. Other days, I needed someone who was also going through the journey to tell me that I wasn't alone and there were days I needed someone to tell me that they were with me and whatever happened, we would face it together.

Going through something so heartbreaking that it affects other peoples' emotions elicits a different response depending upon who is on the receiving end. Depending on the type of relationship I had with the individual, certain circumstances going on in their lives, personality, and past life experiences all contribute to how someone will respond to our story.

The way outsiders, and I say outsiders in a loving way to describe people not affected by a childhood or even adult cancer journey, responded to our family struggles varied greatly. When Cole was first diagnosed, I felt guilty telling people because I didn't want to upset them. Yes, you read that right. When I needed to call the school, tell the boys' coaches, call our pastor, or tell my work, I apologized for what I was experiencing.

This seems so backwards and wrong, but I always look out for others. It's been in my nature as long as I can remember. Even as a child, my goal was to make the world better by helping anyone I could. So, telling someone something that would upset them made me uncomfortable.

I was scared of their reaction because by the way they reacted, I was able to see just how disheartening and scary our situation was and how bad it could become. Seeing how upset others were to hear the news made me face how other people saw what we were going through. It made me feel alone, misunderstood, and completely heartbroken. The way in which the outside world reacted to the trauma we were living elevated the experience and allowed me to see it through a different lens. How I longed to be on the outside, not actually experiencing this nightmare. However, I understood that was not our reality. Wishing it away was not going to change our situation. So, I embraced every moment in the hopes that I could help someone else have an easier journey.

Sometimes I couldn't explain or even understand how people reacted to our story. Instead of acknowledging that it was horrible and offering support, people have said the weirdest things and some of these have jaded me. I became careful of my audience and made sure I was only sharing our story if it was understood. I realized I failed. Sharing with those who understand our story and need to be seen and understood is a necessity, but it is also a necessity to share with those who don't understand and use our story as a teaching moment.

In the beginning, these comments caused me to be cautious and careful in selecting who I shared our story with in order to protect us.

Some things people have said to me are:

"How can you watch your child suffer?"

"I don't understand how you are getting through this."

Or even… "You are living my worst nightmare".

I have actually heard all of these phrases at different points in our journey. The one that kills me is living their worst nightmare. Sometimes I just want to respond with, "yep my worst nightmare too". In those instances where a well-meaning friend says something that makes my skin crawl, I usually remain silent or reply with a generic response like "I know" or in some cases "I don't know".

Facebook is great for these types of comments. Sometimes I don't understand how people think saying these things makes the situation better. In fact, comments like these only made me see the situation in a negative light. These words made the gap between healthy families and our family larger, a cruel reminder that our life was not normal, nor would it ever return to normal. January 15, 2020 was the day we became a childhood cancer family and we will always be a childhood cancer family.

Sometimes words aren't even used. It's the stares and distance like I had a contagious disease and talking to me or getting close to me would ensure they were infected as well. Happening more times than I can tell, when I'm faced with an awkward situation, I just take a deep breath and continue to interact with the person the same way I did prior to diagnosis.

I hope that by teaching others about our journey with pediatric cancer (if they are willing to learn), we will inspire others to join our army and help us advocate for all pediatric cancer patients to have better outcomes, less toxic treatments, and more funding for research and support programs.

Maybe by sharing our story with someone who doesn't understand, I will inspire them to work with the pediatric cancer population or support an organization that helps patients and their families.

By sharing our story with both those who are in our world of pediatric cancer and those who are not a part of this world, I can gain soldiers from two sides of the spectrum to enter the fight and stand tall and proud while supporting, not only us, but others as well.

There is a choice to be made moving forward. We can remain silent and refuse to disclose our experience making our family fit in to the healthy, trauma free existence that constitutes normal in today's society, or we can scream it at the top of our lungs with careless abandon and unwavering advocacy.

I choose the latter. I choose to fight with our warriors, speak up for our survivors, and remember our angels. I will always side with the broken, the fallen, and the brave because I am part of this army, and I will never abandon my fellow warriors.

I will remember those that answered the phone at 1 AM just to listen to me vent and let me know I wasn't alone and I will always pick up the phone for another parent or supporter.

We have to be in this together because if we aren't, the situation is bleak to say the least. There is strength in numbers. There is comfort in pairing with those who understand and have lived through the experience as well. There is support and care in joining a team of childhood cancer advocates, and peace in knowing you are never and will never have to be alone in the fight.

Even though I continue to choose to share our story, it doesn't mean that others keep choosing to listen. And you know what? I'm ok with it. It's part of the journey, and even though we have all lost some friends, we gained even more lifelong friendships along the way.

To further explain the shrinking of our circle of friends, I feel that linking it with simplifying and minimalizing the amount of stuff in one's life is an appropriate analogy. There is something so cathartic in removing clutter and unneeded items from one's life.

I want to switch gears and turn to how I felt going through this experience which explains why I understand the need of others to step away. Since they are not experiencing the trauma first-hand, they have a choice. If it's too painful to hear our story they have the ability to walk away while we do not have that luxury.

As I go through our kitchen and pantry and find outdated, stale, unneeded and unused items and throw them into a lavender scented trash bag, I find relief and a sense of accomplishment in looking at the newly organized and clutter free area. Wouldn't it be amazing if we could do this with our minds? Open the door with a key, like in the *Locke & Key* series. If you haven't heard of this series and have Netflix, it's definitely a good show to pass the time.

In the series, the characters find magic keys and each key allows the user to perform special tasks or have magic abilities. One particular key allows the key holder to walk down the hallway of either their own or someone else's mind and view all the memories they have in storage. By accessing the memories, the key user is able to relive each event as if it were actually happening. Wouldn't it be amazing if we could pick up the thought just like we pick up the clutter of boxes, bowls, and other items that are no longer needed and throw them in a bag that masks their odor and vileness?

If I were able to do this, I would go straight to the aisle holding my anxiety, anxious thoughts, and inner turmoil, pick up the items, and throw them with such a force that takes all my anger, anguish and anxiety and locks it away in a sealed bag to be thrown away forever.

Obviously, this isn't possible. Even with all the advances in technology and healthcare, we cannot control every memory and hardship in the mind. So, managing the trauma and anxiety becomes my next step. I explored finding healthy ways to manage my anxiety and trauma instead of magically ridding my mind of the thoughts forever which is ideal, but impossible. Supporters on the outside have the choice to walk away if it becomes too much. I cannot walk away, but I can employ tools to help manage the turmoil and I have a great support system that continues to make the choice to stay, picking me up when I fall.

As I'm sitting here writing, I'm watching rock music videos, a sweet melody that soothes my thoughts and fuels my fingers with inspiration to type the words on the pages. I mentioned how Cole enjoyed the Foo Fighters when he was younger, and they are one of my favorites as well. The energy that the band exhibits mimics my own, and their words resonate with my soul.

Learning to Walk Again is a video that perfectly describes what I wrote in the previous paragraph. To summarize the video, David Grohl is dealing with some pretty significant stress and encounters people that exasperate the stress and anxiety he is feeling. How does he handle it? Not well, but exactly how I imagine handling such situations if societal norms were not in place.

A convenience store clerk peeves him off, so he hits him with a Slim Jim. Later, some golfers annoy him, so he charges them, steals their golf cart, and runs one of them over. While in a traffic jam, he gets out of his vehicle angrily and just leaves it there in the middle of the other cars, leaving the other drivers wondering what just happened. I absolutely think about doing similar things when my anxiety takes over and I can no longer handle the stress.

It didn't end well for Grohl. He was tased by police while the rest of his band was standing there laughing at the situation. Sometimes, I feel like I've been tased and rendered unconscious by the amount of trauma, anxiety, and stress our family has endured during the past three years which feel like 30. People who were my friends are now just people standing around laughing or paralyzed in total shock at what is going on in my life and no longer good friends, but merely acquaintances that receive a polite hello or wave when seen in public.

They maintain a safe distance in order to protect themselves from the hot mess that is my life. Though cancer is not contagious, in my experience, people behave like it is more contagious than the worst disease imaginable and maybe in the beginning they are supportive and helpful, but as time goes on and things get real, in order to preserve themselves and their sanity, they need to maintain a distance away from the fire. I do not blame them and if I were on the opposite side of the situation, I would most likely do the same to shield myself from the reality and trauma a cancer family will experience.

Even though my friendships are not the same, the few that survived are all I need. In addition to the skeleton crew of long-time friends, I have an army of new friends. We share the trauma, stress, anxiety and life experience of having a child with cancer. These new friends don't run away, steal my golf cart, run me over, or hit me with a Slim Jim. They stand next to me in the fire as I do with them. Shared trauma ensures we understand each other on a level no one can imagine. I can be my authentic self around my warrior mommas. We have all experienced a different level of hell, but can relate in every detail of our stories.

I started to read *The Body Keeps the Score*, a book about trauma, after seeing one of my friends diving into the novel. From the very first pages, I was saying "Oh my goodness, this is all true" and "Wow, yep that's right on the mark". The book describes war veterans and the type of trauma they experienced. Soldiers described in the pages of informative and heartbreaking psychological evidence are more comfortable with others who are part of the group.

In order to get inside, the author needed to become one of them. The veterans made sure he was included by gifting him with a uniform and other gear that ensured he was an insider and able to understand their experience. I have done the same thing. I have sought out moms wearing a gold ribbon pin, bonded with other cancer moms by sharing our stories at events, and connected with a tribe of moms via Zoom through sharing the intimate details of our journey while adorning the same shirts and shrugs signifying to the public that we are warrior moms, and our children are fighters. We are always in this together and even though diagnoses, journeys, and outcomes may differ, we are always bound by the illness that plagued our children and the treatment we all endure.

If you are a mom or supporter of a warrior, know that I understand because I've walked in similar shoes. If you have not experienced such a situation, I do not blame you from distancing yourself from our journey. It is difficult to read, understand, and watch. If you are one of the lucky ones not exposed to this level of terror, I get it.

Watching your child become so sick and endure a treatment that causes even more sickness, is the worst kind of torture I can imagine and that is the reason I will never shut up about pediatric cancer and also the reason we are sharing our story with the world. The rest of the world needs to know the pain in our words to stand up and do something for others in line who may experience this journey in the future.

Cole

My group of friends changed early on in treatment and even though it wasn't because of the cancer, I realize that some people do lose friends through their journey. My closest friends when I was diagnosed are still my friends, but we aren't as close as we were in middle school. They are very supportive and have been throughout my entire journey.

I remember when I was in the PICU, they came and visited me right away. They put on gowns and masks and sat and played video games with me when I was very sick. That's not an easy thing for a teenager to do. Having a friend with cancer is super hard and being the kid with cancer is awful.

I think since everything happened to me when I was a teenager, it was even more difficult. Trying to grow up and be more independent when I didn't have control over anything in my life was hard. My friends didn't have to be as careful about germs, wear masks, and stay away from people like I did.

That was until COVID shut down the world in March of 2020. I was still in the beginning of my treatment. At this point in my journey, I was in consolidation which lasted four months and caused my counts to go low. The quarantine and school from home lasted throughout my difficult parts of treatment. So, I really only missed two months of school before everyone was sent home. This actually helped me to be closer to normal than I would have been had there been no COVID, no masks, and no social distancing.

At this time, students were sent home to do school virtually and everyone needed to wear masks out in public. Sure, I was at the hospital every day and getting chemo, but all my friends were missing out on school, and everyone had to wear masks when they went out in public. So, I didn't feel so different. This really helped. I think it would have been much harder if no one was wearing masks or caring about germs.

Being at home during the hard treatment when I was so tired, and my hair thinned out helped me too. I didn't have to go to school every day, which would be a reminder of how different I felt during that time. Also, my hair never completely fell out, which was really good because I was really worried it would and I didn't want to be bald.

When you go through something really hard in life, you can tell who your true friends are because they are the people that stay behind you no matter what. That's a really hard thing for kids my age because all they should be focused on is being a kid and living their lives. I am grateful my friends and family were concerned for me during treatment and continued to stand beside me as I fought. I feel so proud to have an amazing support system.

Relationships with family and friends can be difficult during normal circumstances. But, throw cancer in there and they become much more difficult. People will come and go, but those that stay are the ones that matter.

Before my diagnosis, I really didn't know what to expect and never even stayed in the hospital overnight. My best friend, Isaiah, did stay in the hospital before, and I remember him telling me what meals I should get when my special diet was finished. His recommendation of the hamburger and staying away from the chicken was a simple tip, but it meant a lot to me. Just remember, your friends and family will do what they can and even the little things are big things and mean a lot.

Even though some of my friends aren't as close with me as they were, I have a really good group of friends and a best friend who does everything with me. I feel like my life is now pretty much back to normal and I'm grateful to be able to hang out with my friends and act like a regular kid. I'm excited to play football this fall and finally get back to normal. I'm no longer embarrassed and don't feel like "the cancer kid". I'm proud to be a survivor.

Just remember, your friends and family will be your biggest cheerleaders and stand next to you every step of the way. Sometimes it's hard for people to be around things that they don't understand, but the people who really deserve you will stay, no questions asked.

CHAPTER 8

Support System
Cancer Is an Enemy Best Fought With an Army

Alone. Such a simple word, but it evokes much fear. Along with fear comes the assumption that all the responsibilities, emotions and consequences are all on you, one single person.

Laura

There is no way I could have gone on this journey alone, although many times during the hell of our experience, I felt very alone. Seeing your child fight for his life is an experience I wouldn't wish on my worst enemy. However, other people who have been on this journey are nowhere near an enemy. They have become my best friends and an amazing support system during our darkest days.

Family has been there for us since day one. They made the proverbial battle shirts that read "Cole Strong," the kind that other cancer families wear with similar phrases to support their warrior and signal to the world that they know an actual real-life superhero. There were fundraisers and donations made in Cole's name to not only support our family, but to throw Cole's name into the bucket of heroes on Earth fighting a formidable enemy.

We were and are very lucky in the fact that both of us were able to keep our jobs, partially thanks to COVID. My husband being deemed an essential employee and my role, switching to remote. My husband, Josh, is one of those people who would go to work under all conditions and illnesses, saving sick days for absolute emergencies.

Prior to COVID, he even went to work unknowingly with the stomach flu and was forced to pull over multiple times on his 20-minute drive home to throw up on the side of the road. Thank goodness no one was following him. I have no clue what they would have thought seeing a grown man throwing up like a carsick toddler all the way home, probably that he was intoxicated and needed to be removed from the road. Needless to say, this earned him a couple of days home recovering with the rest of his sick family who were already contained to the bed with puke buckets and Gatorade on the nightstand.

Since he guarded his sick leave with great care and saved it "just in case," he was able to take the first two months of treatment off to stay with us in the hospital and go to the first clinic visits for chemo.

I was also given this time off because I was set to start my new job three days after Cole was diagnosed. Pushing my start date back allowed me to keep my job the first two months of treatment. COVID and being sent to work from home allowed me to keep my job the remainder of treatment. I often worked out of Cole's hospital room or a quiet, private room the nurses found for me to hold meetings via Zoom. The support of my supervisor during those first few months was never forgotten.

Our pastor, friends from church, Cole's friends, teachers, and coworkers all rallied behind us in the fight. Those very first months, the support that we received was amazing. Gift baskets and home visits from an amazing teacher, an amazing classmate of Cole's who organized a kickball tournament, donations from a fire company and little pick-me-up gifts and cards from family and friends were our lifeline through diagnosis and treatment when we were still in shock and so numb.

I have often heard that comparison is the killer of joy, and the next statement I am going to type embodies that thought. Comparing our journey to the journey of other local warriors and seeing the widespread, community and public support of these fighters and comparing it to our own small and private circle makes me think "Why is their fight any different than ours?" "Why do they get a ton of support and a large army backing them and we don't have the same type of support?"

Well, I can answer these questions quite simply. The reason why our fight wasn't so public and we didn't have the entire school rallying behind us or huge fundraisers supporting our warrior is because our circle is small but mighty. I have always kept a small circle of loyal friends and our family, as a whole, has always been a private family. We guard our experiences and keep many things to ourselves simply because we like it that way and get overwhelmed with too much attention. I have always been this way since I was a child, and Cole also has this trait. We wanted it like this to preserve whatever was remaining of our sanity and be able to breathe and go through the motions of our nightmare.

It's important to realize every family is different. Every fight is different. Every response is different. Give the family grace and take their cues. I may look back and think "why did this family have so much support," but, then I realize we made the choice to have a small but mighty presence of supporters because it's what helped us through the fight to prevent overwhelm and burnout. If I pushed people away, it was because cancer sucks. It's hard and awful and full of darkness.

Having too many things going on contributed to more stress than I could fit in my bucket. The proverbial bucket I'm talking about was full and overflowing with trauma, side effects, stress, hospitalizations, chemo reactions, and appointments, and I couldn't add anything else to the bucket without completely losing my mind. We did what we had to do to survive.

However, when things progressed and it seemed like Cole was having reaction after reaction and multiple hospitalizations earned us frequent stay points in the oncology floor member reward system, the support faded to the background. At a time when we needed someone to vent to and encourage us to keep going, it was harder to find someone to offer support. Our family was always there because that's what our family does. We love and support one another in any situation.

However, others seemed to sink into the wall at the high school dance with all the other wallflowers and no longer danced with us in our trauma and heartache. Our trauma became too much for them to continue to carry and to preserve their mental health and sanity or for reasons unknown to us they bowed out.

The people who stayed on the dance floor - guess who they were? They were survivors. Either they personally experienced cancer or supported someone very close to them going through the fight. They knew the choreography to the dance by heart and continued to hold our hand as we gained our footing after each stumble.

Not only did the survivors stay, but obviously so did Cole's medical team who volunteered to expose themselves to the experience of childhood cancer as a profession. The doctors, nurses, surgeons, child life specialists, and social workers supported us while we were at the hospital because it was their job. Even though they go home at the end of the day and resume their normal lives, I know they carry the patients and families with them everywhere they go. I give them so much credit because for some reason or another, the choice was made to expose themselves daily to the heartache, trauma, hell, and death that is pediatric cancer. Making themselves vulnerable to heartache allows them to help people like our family and guide us through our journey.

When I was in graduate school, one of my professors who I hold to a high regard shared with the class that many, if not all PSY.D (Psychology Doctorate) candidates are required to participate in individual therapy as a condition of their program. The reasoning behind this stipulation is the belief backed by science that a clinician is only able to take their patient as far into the depths of their mind as they are willing to go themselves. This belief helps me to understand a lot of things. One of those things is the reason why many of our supporters chose to fade into the background. The conclusion I could come up with is they reached their limit. In order to preserve themselves and their well-being, they chose to not go as far into the darkness as we were being forced to endure. We did not have a choice. Neither did other survivors and fighters. The magic key that allows you to pick and choose which experiences stay in your brain does not exist so there are no quick fixes.

I'm also brought back to this thought while writing our story. I can only share as deep as I am willing to re-experience. In order to give you the full, impossible and heartbreaking at times but also miraculous and inspiring story, I have to re-experience every heartache, every chest pain, and every short breath all over again.

Sometimes I feel like I'm right there in the hospital or clinic reliving the hell, until I actually open my eyes from the dream and realize I'm safely on my chair with my dog typing away on the keyboard in front of me. The inner turmoil and unrest are completely worth the pain if our story is able to help others who share a similar experience before or after our own journey.

I am forever grateful to the fighters and survivors who chose to fight along with us, surely re-experiencing their own heartache along the way. That's the thing about childhood cancer. It's terrible and heart-wrenching, something you never want to experience or watch someone else experience, but the moment someone else is forced to live this hell, it's like a siren only pediatric cancer families can hear is blaring, beckoning us all to stand on the frontlines. As soon as the siren utters its sound, I'm there with all my armor and weapons and I will fight along other warriors every step of the way.

During the intense parts of chemo, not only did we isolate ourselves from others due to COVID and germs in general that could make Cole very sick, but I noticed that I isolated myself from other parents in the fight to an extent. In the beginning, I kept my distance from supporters and kept our circle small, but as we progressed through treatment and I found the capacity to add more to our circle, I was very selective in who and what I allowed to enter our space.

I had to reach out to others on my terms. Any additional information or heartache could push me to the brink of collapse, and I could not risk not being able to be there for my son. Once the strong chemo was over and the side effects were much less severe and spread out in nature, I felt it was safe to expand my network without being so vulnerable. This is not to say I didn't reach out to others for support previously. I did. However, I didn't fully immerse myself in support groups and nonprofit organizations to connect and help others in the fight until about a year into Cole's treatment. Prior to maintenance, we were in the thick of things and anxiety was the Tasmanian Devil ripping through everything in my mind and causing panic. The point when Cole was about to enter the maintenance phase gave me enough breathing room to reach out for a hand to hold and also give my hand for support at the same time.

I found tremendous support and healing in Momcology® which is a nonprofit organization comprised of moms and caregivers supporting children who currently or previously had cancer. Since we were about a year into COVID-19 when I was given the opportunity to attend a retreat with other moms, it was held virtually.

The online delivery did not decrease the effectiveness of the tools I was given, or the relationships made through our weekend experience. I picked the perfect time to join, but that doesn't mean it wasn't difficult at times. When anyone was going through a hospitalization or crisis with their child, I felt it as well.

I was walking along with them in their journey while trying to keep the footing in our own. The benefits far outweighed the risks. The sisterhood we shared, the people I met through the experience, and the mental tools I was given to manage the stress and anxiety and ease the trauma were beyond what I could ever imagine.

During the retreat experience, we were all given several meaningful packages. The first gift we received was a shrug, a crocheted "hug" given to cancer moms, adorned in maroon and purple thread with a gold tie. Seeing all the moms on screen each wearing their shrug solidified the thought that we are all in this together.

Draped by identical material and wearing our hearts on our sleeves, we embarked on a truly transformational experience. I cannot express the amount of gratitude I have for this organization. No one can or should fight this battle alone. If COVID-19 taught me only one thing, it is that I cannot thrive in isolation and crave the company and support of others but on my own terms. I am complicated. What can I say? Being alone or feeling alone in the fight is beyond terrifying. I never want to feel hopeless or as if we are the only family experiencing heartache.

Just knowing a community of moms exists within my connections and are available any day or time I'm in need, puts my heart at ease. I like the phrase "there is strength in numbers" because it's true. If you are fighting a huge battle by yourself and the other side has an enormous army of soldiers, the likelihood you will survive very long is slim.

Mental or physical exhaustion will occur almost immediately as the other side wins. If you are surrounded and supported by an army that is the same size, the battle may be difficult, but the chance of winning is much better. Now, if you were supported by a fierce, aggressive, army of passionate moms that outnumbers the army in physical presence and strength, you will win regardless of the difficulty or duration of the battle.

The amazing support of a fierce tribe of warrior moms is just the thing I needed to help pull me out of the pit of despair and prevent me from feeling like all hope was lost when I was overrun by our journey and just plain tired and stressed.

When the waves kept coming and side effects kept happening or we had an unexpected hospitalization or illness, my mom tribe stood up and stopped the waves long enough for me to catch my breath.
Pediatric cancer families are easy to spot because we are passionate, sometimes if not most of the time loud and exuberant, fierce and often seen wearing gold or a specific diagnosis color like orange for leukemia.

Sometimes I feel like a Jeep owner or motorcycle rider who has code signals to other Jeep owners or motorcycle riders when I see someone wearing cancer gear, a pediatric cancer T-shirt or organization gear supporting anything related to the cause. I want to yell out, "Me too, we are in the journey too, I'm with you". Obviously, I don't do that, or at least I think I've never yelled at complete strangers, but I feel seen and supported and have a need to yell back my support to let the wearer know they are not alone.

When the crisis mode subsided and I was no longer fighting to keep it together while offering support to my child who was literally fighting for each moment, I had this unrelenting need to help others in our situation. I felt extremely lucky that we both had our jobs. No one had to make the choice of employment or staying with Cole and we didn't have any huge medical or other expenses rendering us paralyzed.

We were doing well enough to forgo financial resources and leave funds for those who truly needed assistance. All things considered, we had jobs, we didn't have huge expenses or hardships like flying thousands of miles or driving hours to treatment, so I consider it a win in the general life category.

Since we didn't need such resources, I was extremely moved by others who experienced such hardships and wanted to do everything in my power to help make it a little easier on families. No one should have to watch their child battle cancer, but those of us who are unlucky enough to not have a choice, should absolutely NOT have to choose between supporting our child or paying bills. So, I wanted to help others who needed me or someone like me who understood what they were going through on a level someone who never experienced a child with cancer cannot.

When we were first admitted, a social worker came into our room with a stack of papers instructing us how to apply for medical assistance. I was taken aback because I didn't want to reach out to anyone, let alone the state for help. I was raised in a family who believed you should never take help from someone else and instead help others in any way possible.

Further explanation eased my worry because in our state, Pennsylvania, children with serious and long-term illnesses qualified for medical assistance without the usual financial stipulation and the limits are extremely high.

In our case, it helped with copays and the countless prescriptions we filled on a weekly basis amongst other things. After explaining many of the resources available to us in addition to medical assistance, the social worker handed me a flyer for ThinkBIG® Pediatric Cancer Fund.

Since our treating hospital was only a few miles from our home and this organization actually resided in our town, I was familiar with them because I've seen the amazing things they did in our community. So months later, my mind returned to that social worker and her flyer. I reached out to the founder of ThinkBIG® and spewed out my story in an email. I asked him how I could help.

I must have taken him by surprise since I was a family in the fight and I was not asking for help, but I was asking to help others. After making sure I didn't need assistance, the president and his manager met with me via Zoom to hear what I could offer the organization. After a 20-minute Zoom meeting, I was asked to consider taking an open board position, had an interview scheduled with current board members, and wrote a list of things I wanted to accomplish.

Fast forward a few months, I was not only on the board, but I am currently the organization's secretary. The year and a half of membership with such an amazing organization has allowed me to give back, but not only that, it has given me support in ways I never thought I needed.

This group of people is the kindest and among the most caring individuals I have ever met. Sure, some of them have experienced pediatric cancer, but not all are in the fight. They chose to help on their own accord and through their choice, I found support and encouragement and bottled some of it up to give to others.

I have been able to fill the desire to help others and give back to a community who picked me up and held me together when I was experiencing the worst trauma of my life. I am able to use my degree in School Counseling to brainstorm programming and events for pediatric cancer patients and their families. I am able to offer social and emotional support to families while advocating for others and screaming the issues so many of us feel at one point or another during this journey.

Yes, there are times when I choose to be private and keep to myself, but Cole's diagnosis and journey has exposed me to a level of trauma I never knew existed. I wasn't given a choice. Neither was Cole.

Therefore, we understand others do not choose this absolutely heart-wrenching, vile disease. For some reason, I will never understand why cancer chooses us. I believe with my whole heart that God is walking before us and sees what we, as humans, cannot see. Therefore, He knows the outcome and clears the path. Everything happens according to His plan and for reasons I do not know, all the pieces aligned to allow me to give back and soothe the burning desire to make it even just a little bit easier for others who have no choice but to fight.

Many times, throughout our journey, I questioned myself and I questioned why this happened to Cole. I looked for signs telling me I'm on the right path and things will turn out ok. I've screamed and yelled to God to show me signs and although He always responds in His time with undeniable signs, sometimes it's just downright hard.

When I chose to become involved with ThinkBIG Pediatric Cancer Fund, I knew almost immediately I was on the right path. I experienced several signs letting me know I am supposed to support this organization. When I first met the founder and manager, I realized the manager was from my hometown, just like one of Cole's nurses. Little did I know, the manager graduated high school with my cousin Jessie, and our fathers worked together. My parents knew his family well and we work together like we've known each other most of our lives. The support, work ethic, and willingness to help others is evident in every fundraiser, event, or activity of the organization.

Having an army of support is not an easy or simple process and there is no rhyme or reason in choosing your army and who you let be a part of your journey. I found when I am in tune with myself and what our family needs as a whole, I am able to clearly advocate for the type of support we need.

If someone offers to join you in the fight and you are comfortable in allowing them to share in the good, bad, and ugly of the journey, do it. Remember, cancer is a battle best fought with an army. The size and strength of the soldiers in the army are important to the overall success in the battle. A good support system goes a long way and may preserve what is left of our sanity and ease some of the anxiety when general overwhelming feelings or confusion come into play.

Cole

No one can or should have to go through a cancer journey alone. The best way to win a war is with a strong army behind you. I am proud to say that I have a very supportive family, group of friends, and even strangers who all rallied together and encouraged me during different parts of my journey.

When I was first diagnosed, it was before COVID began and I was able to have visitors in the hospital. My family and friends all came to cheer me on and encourage me as I started my fight. My two best friends came to visit and played video games with me which distracted me from everything going on at the time. My brother and my grandparents also came multiple times to check on me and show me they were there for me. My uncle, knowing I love history and WWII in particular, had a leather jacket with a map and WWII scene printed inside. He knew I would love it and brought it to my house when I was discharged from the hospital. I still have it and look at it often, remembering his kindness.

My parents stayed in the hospital the entire time and never left. Each time I was hospitalized, one of my parents was always right by my side. I liked having them with me, but sometimes it was difficult always being with people and never having a moment to be alone. There was always someone in my hospital room, whether it was visitors, family, or my doctors and nurses.

When I got home and I was able to be alone, it was both nice and scary.

By myself, I was able to really think about what was going on and let the fact that I had cancer and was facing a long road of treatment sink in. I enjoyed having the company for many reasons and it was a great distraction.

When COVID started and I couldn't have visitors, I was still able to connect with my friends on social media and online when we played our video games. I didn't feel as alone because everyone was at home and in the same situation. It definitely felt a lot different though, because not as many people were coming and going from my room. In the quiet and alone, the time seemed to go a lot slower.

When I was in the hospital or in the clinic, there was another huge team of fighters by my side. All my nurses, doctors, child life specialists and everyone else at the hospital were very helpful and supportive. They fought along my side from the very first day and even now during my appointments and check-ups. It really meant so much to me and made me feel comfortable to know that my team was so attentive.

Outside of the hospital, my teachers at the time that I was diagnosed, all wrote me cards and showed me that they were behind me and supporting me. One of my friends even held a dodgeball tournament for me at our school and the entire school played dodgeball in my honor.

My aunt had T-shirts made that were black with orange writing because the awareness color for leukemia is orange. They said, "Cole Strong" and everyone wore them to support me which meant a lot to me and showed that they cared.

Sometimes I got really overwhelmed with everything that was going on. It was almost always in those moments when I was overwhelmed and filled with anxiety, that someone would check on me and make sure I was doing ok. I was shocked by all the support and honored that they would take the time to make sure I was ok and cared that I was going through this battle.

Not only did people I knew and lived close to support me, but people I met because of this journey that lived far away did as well. One of these people is another fighter, Molly Oldham, who battled brain cancer… twice. She was asked to sing the National Anthem at a Florida Panthers game multiple times.

Molly is super talented and has a great voice. During the Hockey Fights Cancer game, she sang, and everyone made signs naming who they fight against cancer for. I never met Molly in person. My mom knows her mom, but Molly put my name on a sign among other fighters and that meant so much. We never met. She didn't know who I was or anything about me besides the fact that I was fighting leukemia and thought enough to include me in her support.

That's the thing with this "cancer club." No one ever wants to be a part of it, and everyone hates when someone new comes to the club, but because they understand exactly what you are going through, each person will support the other as much as possible. Knowing there are thousands of people around the world supporting you is an amazing feeling, but the battle is tough and cannot be done alone.

CHAPTER 9

Benched During Your Prime
Struggles Unique to Teens

The teenage years are an awkward, cranky few years of turmoil resulting in one step closer to adulthood and independence in more than one way.

Laura

Imagine being told you have a life-threatening disease such as cancer and going into the hospital or clinic and everything is child-sized. Think about Alice in Wonderland and the mushroom the caterpillar gives Alice that instantly turns her into a giant. The looming figure of Alice towers over the furniture and even the houses and other structures in Wonderland. I believe, at one point, Alice might even break some furniture or cause some other type of havoc on the little land beneath her feet.

Of course, this is a huge exaggeration as fairytales and cartoons often are in order to get and keep our attention, but not too far from the truth of a teen entering a clinic designed for much smaller beings. The chairs in the waiting rooms are small, the exam tables are short, and the reclining chairs in the clinic room are also minuscular. Toys are placed on shelves or in bins in the waiting room (prior to COVID) and everything is decorated in bright colors and with child-friendly designs like animals and cartoons.

Imagine Alice again, in a foreign area like Wonder Land resembling a fish out of water or a giant in a much smaller habitat. Teens have outgrown the furnishings and decorations in Pediatric Clinic Land and may feel out of place, like things were not designed with our teen patients in mind. They weren't.

Since the majority of patients are much smaller, the design of pediatric hospitals including the clinic areas are aimed at making the tiniest patients comfortable so they don't feel like Alice when she ate the mushroom that made her shrink into a miniature version of herself with huge furniture, treatment tables and stark white walls.

It really is like Wonderland and the changes Alice experiences. The smallest patients will feel smaller if things aren't their size and the largest patients will feel even larger trying to squeeze into small equipment.

In designing a clinic based upon the need of the majority, the minority is overlooked. In an ideal world, one or two rooms, one or two chairs, and one or two shelves will be set aside for our teen patients allowing this overlooked population to be seen and accounted for in every aspect of their care. Knowledge, understanding, and of course, funding are common reasons for not including both populations in one area.

There are several things that need to be considered when serving two very different populations. Let's begin with knowledge. If you are the parent of a warrior, you know exactly what I am talking about regarding the furnishings and decor because you have likely tried to fit your butt in a child-sized chair or bent down to reach the child-sized table. Parents adapting to such furniture and equipment is very similar to a teenage boy the size of Cole (who is way larger than me, by the way) attempting to fit into small furniture and adapt to an environment he outgrew five plus years ago.

I understand the majority of the patients using the furniture and equipment are the appropriate size for such objects, but one important and often overlooked population is teenagers who are much larger, and the furnishings should match their stature as well. This patient demographic is slighted in more ways than imaginable.

Everything is geared towards children and not many things are aimed at the teenage population. Feeling out of place is an understatement. I still remember the very first time we went to the clinic after Cole was discharged from his initial hospital stay. We were ushered into a waiting room with four child-sized recliners along the wall, a child-sized table with four child-sized kitchen chairs in the middle, and one lone adult rocking chair (which was broken by the way). The funny part is the rocker was most likely placed for adults to sit on and rock their baby or toddler, not for a teenage patient to have an appropriate piece of furniture upon which to relax.

The wall on the far side was covered in colorful locked boxes, each holding toys, play dough, craft supplies and other objects geared toward children. A dirty toy bin laid on the floor filled with action figures, dolls, and other toys used by patients prior to our arrival. The TV on the wall was playing cartoons and colorful drawings and crafts adorned the opposite wall. The room looked like a preschool classroom or daycare center taking care of elementary school aged or even younger children, not teenagers.

Of course, the only normal sized piece of furniture was that rocker and it was taken by a parent rocking a very small child so Cole was forced to squeeze into one of the mini recliners while my husband and I opted to stand and wait for normal furniture in the clinic room. Oh, how we hoped for a normal sized chair to sit on and rest. However, I'll be uncomfortable every single day of treatment if that means my child can have the appropriate place to be a little more comfortable and at ease during a harrowing experience of receiving chemotherapy.

One unique detail regarding our treating hospital lies in the design of the clinic. Most oncology clinics have an infusion room lined with multiple treatment chairs where patients sit while hooked up to poison that is pumped through their veins. Our clinic is small and has a much different layout. The waiting room described above is the first room in the hallway painted institutional white.

The next five rooms are treatment rooms. Our patients do not go to an infusion room. Each patient has their own exam room with two chairs, a recliner (most likely child-sized) and an exam table. I was incredible grateful to be in a room to ourselves, especially when we needed to occupy the clinic for eight plus hours in one day.

Even though each family had a private room, the room itself was small and every time we came for treatment, the nurses complained of the size and layout which certainly made it difficult to move around quickly and limited the number of medical professionals who could be present at one time.

Our medical staff was very attentive to Cole and incredibly thoughtful. Since we basically lived at the hospital the first nine plus months of treatment and the staff knew our visits were long and frequent, we were always given room five, the only room with the normal sized recliner.

Cole preferred to receive his chemotherapy in the reclining chair rather than on the exam table because the table was entirely too short for his five-foot six-inch body and a good deal of his legs hung off the edge even when the foot rest was extended. Since we were seen multiple times a week, staff knew Cole's preference to sit in the adult sized recliner and reserved our room. One nurse even called it the "Cole Suite" and said we should have a plaque made to hang right outside the door designating it as such.

In addition to mini furniture and decor aimed at a much younger population, Cole experienced a difference in the type of support he received. No, not in medical care. Our medical team was amazing and provided great care. I am describing child life services and other emotional/social support and programs outside of the hospital.

Cole did not receive the same type or frequency of support as the younger population of patients (that was until the amazing child life specialist Rose came to clinic). I discussed this with Rose as she tried to come up with support to offer teenage patients. The care Cole received from Rose, first in Pediatric Sedation and then in the clinic, was amazing. She really does provide equal support to all patients when possible. She went out of her way to get Cole the perfect end of treatment gift, a basketball, a balloon, and his favorite type of cookie cake presenting him with everything during our bell ringing ceremony. Prior to her, there was minimal to no support, and it was obvious the teenage patients were left out. I absolutely do not blame the previous child life specialist. The teenage population is difficult to support which is why I'm making it my mission to provide the type of support relevant to teenagers and aid hospitals in utilizing programs, organizations, and items beneficial to teens receiving treatment.

Yes, it's easier to give younger patients a toy or stuffed animal to provide comfort and show you care but, you know what? Sometimes that is what Cole wanted as well. Even before Rose came to clinic, she was in the pediatric sedation department where we would frequently visit for spinal taps. We will never ever forget her kindness and the attention she placed on making sure Cole was comfortable and seen. On holidays, Cole was offered a specific holiday Ty Beanie Baby. He always accepted. So, we have multiple Valentine's Day, St. Patrick's Day, and patriotic beanie bears lining Cole's shelf. We always seemed to land in pediatric sedation on a holiday.

Not only did this amazing person treat Cole just the same as her younger patients, but she made a huge deal about the time prior to when Cole fell asleep (he was sedated during spinal taps) which is nerve-racking and anxiety provoking for some patients.

She put Cole at ease and joked non-stop saying she was going to style his thinning hair. Really, it wasn't a bluff, she actually did braid, clip and ponytail his hair. I believe there was even a headband or two in the mix. We saved all the hair supplies and thanks to her, I now have a pretty decent supply of pictures to show Cole's future wife or bribe him to do his chores.

Cole went along with everything and honestly, it lightened the mood and showed Cole that he had support at every corner. I often rolled Cole back into the clinic in a wheelchair with a great new hairstyle, putting a huge smile on the nurses and doctors' faces and brightening the gloomy mood of a serious hallway.

Other than our amazingly compassionate child life specialist who wears her heart on her sleeve and shows up for her patients, even coming to his last home track meet, the support was noticeably less than our younger patients. Though the younger population absolutely needs the attention and distraction, the teenagers do as well. Even if they seem more adult-like, they are still children in a very key developmental stage and should be approached and cared for appropriately.

A teenage boy the size of a grown man may not seem like he would want a stuffed animal or coloring book, but how will you know if you don't ask? Offering the stuffed animal, craft, coloring book or toy is better than ignoring the patient altogether. Finding age-appropriate resources for teenagers going through treatment is a goal of ours and we hope to provide hospitals and patients with items and learning materials based not only on Cole's experience, but other patients as well.

Many items work for all ages and can be donated to your local children's hospital for the older patients. Items such as ear buds, art supplies, coloring materials, board games, playing cards and card games, fuzzy socks, or blankets are absolutely age-appropriate gifts and should bring a smile to a patient who may not be used to receiving extra attention.

Supporting the teenage patient population is extremely difficult because the stage of development in the teenage years is categorized by several very important tasks. During this stage of development, a child prepares for adulthood assuming not only a physical appearance resembling an adult but acquires adult-like responsibilities and asserts their independence from parents and caregivers.

In addition to becoming independent and asserting their capability, teens also have an important role with their same age peers. To successfully move through adolescence, teenagers need to be accepted by their peers and be included in a group of friends. Maturing socially, physically, and emotionally are also part of the great teenage experience.

Understanding adolescent development, although it sounds like the name of a television show, is pivotal to developing a support program for teenage patients in and out of the hospital environment. My hope in giving you a mini developmental psychology lesson is to create an understanding of important issues to teens to provide insight and clarity as to the type of initiatives beneficial to the adolescent/young adult population of patients.

Mini lesson takeaway involves becoming independent and assuming more adult-like responsibilities. Teens may want to be completely involved in their treatment and care. I am of the firm belief that this is extremely important, but I understand that many people may have varying opinions in the matter. Each child is different, and parents should be tuned into what they believe their child is capable of handling at each moment.

My husband and I kept Cole involved from the very beginning. We did not sugarcoat or keep anything from him from diagnosis day on. I never want him to look back and say "why didn't you tell me", or have any type of regret during his treatment. Cole was and is involved in every decision. I do realize that it is a ton for any person to handle, let alone a teenager who is trying so hard to find themselves, grow, and develop into an adult, but it was our decision and the right one for our family.

Including Cole in every decision was a lot, but I wouldn't change it if I had to go back in time. I believe we made the correct decision for our child who, as a result, is very informed regarding his health, medical care, and possible long-term side effects. I need to give credit to Cole's medical team who may be used to treating young children, but certainly do extremely well with teenage patients, keeping Cole informed and a primary participant of the journey from day one.

No one should ever have to go on such a traumatic journey, but Cole's path has certainly prepared him for adulthood in an "everything is on fire" kind of way. Though traumatic, Cole made decisions very few teenagers have to face.

Making the extremely difficult decisions with us prepared him for making any type of decision in the future such as which college to attend, what occupation to pursue, and what kind of car to buy. It's extremely important to consider the child's developmental phase when making decisions, not solely in a cancer patient role, but in everyday life as well. Cole has always been a very mature, quiet soul and with his parents and medical team at his side, we guided him along the way.

Another developmental tidbit to keep in the forefront is the importance of peers in a teen's life. Peer relationships are some of the most important relationships adolescents and teenagers have because they play a huge role in their emotional and social development, and how these relationships grow and develop directly impacts later developmental stages. Teens look to their peers for approval and acceptance during this stage. Fitting in and being just one of the group is extremely important.

A teenager going through cancer treatment will not always fit in. Hair loss is the main characteristic that will set a cancer patient apart from the rest of the teens in a group. I distinctly remember Cole telling us in the PICU when he was first admitted and very sick that he "did not want to undergo chemo if he was going to lose his hair".

Forget, being nauseous, losing or gaining weight, being admitted to the hospital, not being able to go to school and not being able to participate in all the things his friends were doing, the hair loss would make him stand out like a sore thumb. I believe some of the thoughts going through his mind were related to the fact that he could hide his battle for the most part, but when his hair was gone and he looked the part of a cancer patient, he needed to fully embody the role and come to terms with his cancer battle.

He would no longer be one of the crowd and fitting in would be near impossible. Hair and appearance were a huge concern and preoccupation at this stage in his life as a middle schooler in the beginning of treatment and a high schooler for the remainder of his journey.

Recognizing adolescent developmental stages is helpful to understanding where your child resides in emotional and social development and what parts of the battle may be extremely difficult. Loss of hair may be something very difficult for adults as well, but for different reasons.

Cole was one of the "lucky ones". He never completely lost his hair. Yes, it thinned a lot, but it was still there. His oncologist couldn't believe he retained some of his gorgeous locks and remembered only one or two patients in his 20 plus years equally as lucky.

Undergoing treatment during the COVID-19 pandemic was a blessing in some ways. Even though it was an awful and isolating time in the world, it leveled the playing field for Cole during treatment. Since everyone was required to wear masks and isolate, our family did not feel like we stuck out like we would have if the world was normal for the majority of our treatment.

I still remember going to the grocery store at the beginning of Cole's treatment and wearing a mask because I didn't want to expose Cole to any germs. I stuck out, completely. Since this was January or February 2020 before COVID protocols were in place and masks were not required; I felt awkward. I couldn't even imagine a teenager wearing a mask in public, let alone school during a normal time.

Also, since we were isolated and sent to the safety of our homes, the blow of missing school and opportunities to hang out with friends was lessened. Everyone was isolated, online for school, and forbidden to socialize. Since Cole is the kid who never wants to stand out and tends to blend into the crowd, never causing waves, this worked to our advantage in a terrible situation.

Part of the reason Cole and I decided to write a book is to shine the light on this often-hidden population of pediatric cancer patients. The in-between stage of not a child any longer but, not yet an adult, is awkward but extremely important in developmental terms. Having the correct supports in place for this population of patients can directly impact their experience and make a huge difference in a very important developmental phase. I understand I placed emphasis on having the right sized furniture, medical equipment and appropriate decor and it may seem trivial, but these seemingly little things can make an out-of-place teenage patient feel seen and understood in a foreign land. At least when Alice was the same size as the other characters in Wonderland, she didn't feel so out of place.

Cole

When I was diagnosed, I never thought that it would happen to me. I knew I didn't feel well, but I never thought that I had cancer. I really didn't know anything about cancer or even know anyone who fought the disease. The only things that I was thinking about in 8th grade were working out, staying in shape for football, and getting to go to high school the next year and play junior varsity football. I didn't think that I would be in the hospital fighting for my life and spending so much time in the hospital and clinic getting chemo. The cancer treatment took over every aspect of my life and I couldn't do anything without making sure it was ok and wasn't going to make me sick or have to go into the hospital.

I learned a lot about my treatment and way more about medical things than any teenager should ever need to know. I was constantly thinking about my cancer, and I couldn't wait to be finished with treatment so I could get back to a normal life. It felt like my life was on pause for three years and I couldn't do anything that didn't involve my treatment.

I didn't understand why this was happening to me and why I couldn't just be a kid and not be worried about germs hurting me, the chemo side effects or spending day after day in the hospital getting poked and different types of tests and medicine.

I was really worried about losing my hair as I said before. I liked my hair and couldn't imagine what I would look like if I didn't have any hair. I don't really like wearing hats, so I never really covered my head. I just let my thinning hair alone and was lucky it never all fell out. When I got to maintenance, my hair came back super curly and my oncologist and I used to compare who had the bigger, curlier hair. The doctors and nurses called this "chemo curl". The months of intense chemotherapy can often cause the hair that comes back during the maintenance stage of treatment to have a curl. When my hair started to grow back, I noticed it was getting curly. Within a couple of months, my entire head was filled with curls. Though they only stayed a year or two, it was neat to see such a difference in the way my hair looked. From talking to other cancer patients, some said they kept curls or their hair grew back darker or lighter. Even though I didn't keep my curls, my hair is a bit darker than it was before treatment.

Yes, I was very worried about my hair and appearance, but I had a bigger task at hand. I needed to get through this battle. I was climbing a large mountain and it certainly wasn't easy. However, I knew the view at the top of the mountain would be beautiful. I just needed to get through the difficult parts of the trek to get to the view at the top.

Being a teenager in the pediatric clinic and in the children's hospital was awkward. Everything was so small, including all the recliners and chairs in the rooms. There were toys everywhere and the little kids made crafts and played games. I was bored a lot during the long treatment days, but there was really nothing for a teenager to do except play on my phone, nap, or watch movies.

I want to start an organization for teenage cancer patients that connects them to their favorite sports teams by sending them team gear like shirts and balls. Sports are a big part of my life and I was able to connect with a couple of organizations that did this for me. It really helped on my hard days. Since there aren't really any organizations for teenagers, I want to help some day and make it easier for other patients.

Being a teenager in treatment is hard in many ways. It felt like nothing was made for me and I didn't really belong in the children's hospital, but I didn't feel like I belonged in the main hospital either. It was also hard because I understood everything that was happening. Some things were confusing and scary, but everyone on my team did a really good job at explaining things so that I would understand.

Understanding everything was difficult because it caused my anxiety to get worse and I worried about every little thing. I can see how it was hard for the younger patients because they didn't understand what was happening to them but sometimes, I think that would be easier. I was aware of everything and understood everything that was going on and knew what I was missing out on in life.

I couldn't play football because of the port, and I missed three seasons of a sport I love. Also, I love to swim and used to go to the creek with friends before diagnosis which I could no longer do. I was able to swim in my pool and my friend's pool, but no public pools, oceans, waterparks, or creeks. Not being able to do things that my friends were doing and feeling like I was holding them back was very difficult.

I believe there needs to be more support for teenagers because there are many teenage patients, and I don't believe they get as many services as the younger patients. It's such a hard time to go through a cancer diagnosis because all I wanted to do was be a kid and I couldn't because everything was controlled and my entire life revolved around my treatment.

Supporting teenagers is very important because they don't fit into either of the big groups of patients like kids or adults. I was in between both age groups, so supports and techniques from either group could work and should be looked into to make sure the patients feel comfortable and supported.

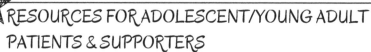

RESOURCES FOR ADOLESCENT/YOUNG ADULT PATIENTS & SUPPORTERS

Bite me Cancer

Teen Cancer America (teencanceramerica.org/news-resources)

Make-A-Wish ®

Love your Melon

Cancer Care

Jessie Rees Foundation - NEGU and JoyJars (www.negu.org)

Cancer for College

Project Outrun

Elephants and Tea

ThinkBIG® Pediatric Cancer Fund- Pennsylvania residents only

18 Loop- VR for Teens with Cancer (www.18loop.org)

CHAPTER 10

Healing From the Journey

$\mathcal{E}$motional trauma is something that needs to be treated just like physical disease.

Laura

Things that occur during the teenage stage of development can follow someone through young adulthood and even into their adult years.

Trauma occurring during this stage of development can set the stage for additional mental health struggles later in life.

Since I am bearing my soul in this book already, I want to share an experience that occurred in my teenage developmental stage, having a negative impact on my emotional, mental health, and self-image, even now.

Whatever your family dynamic may be, there always seems to be that one family member that you connect with on a much deeper level than anyone else. For you, it may be a sibling, a parent, grandparent, aunt or uncle. This special person may not even be a family member at all. Maybe it's your spouse, best friend, or someone else in your life. For me, it was my Grammy Carol, my dad's mom.

As I type this, I feel the smile pull on my face and my heart swelling with the pride of being her granddaughter. Amazing, intelligent, giving, and caring are all words used to describe my Grammy, but none of them give justice to her amazing soul and the bond we shared. I gravitated towards her house of hidden treasures like a magnet to a piece of metal. Since my Pap died when I was seven, she lived alone, and I aimed to fill the solitude and void of loneliness by being with her as much as possible.

I soaked in all the stories and advice she offered like a sponge drinking the purest water. I spent hours each day during the summer just exploring her house, listening to her stories, watching the birds from her window and eating Stella Dora cookies which are amazing vanilla and chocolate Italian cookies that I ate plain or often dunked in milk. I liked the vanilla more than the chocolate and often picked these out of the package, leaving my Grammy with a plastic tray full of chocolate flavored goodness. I still hold those memories close to my heart and cherish the time I had with the most amazing woman I've ever met.

I realize now, that spending time with my grandmother allowed me to be closer to my dad who I only saw on weekends or the occasional day I went to his house during the week. When I was with my Grammy, I felt closer to my dad, and he was often at her house too so I was able to see him even more.

My grandmother had diabetes and a heart condition and wasn't in the best of health. She was in her late sixties when she had a diabetic episode that she described as "someone picking her up and throwing her to the floor". At that point, she could not move, the loss of feeling in her hands and legs immediately evident. My dad was always the one out of four children she called in emergencies due to close proximity and trust. So, when the ambulance company called my dad, he immediately went to the hospital. After receiving a battery of tests, pokes, and prods, it was determined my grandmother suffered from diabetic neuropathy which is a loss of feeling in the extremities due to long-term effects of diabetes. The doctors were not sure if the feeling would return and suggested she enter a nursing facility to ensure she had the proper care.

My unlimited visits and time spent wandering through the comfort of my grandmother's home were over as she was transitioned to a nursing home about 45 minutes away. Distance did not stop the visits, and my dad and I went at least two times a week to spend time with her.

She quickly became accustomed to her temporary (she always knew she would return to her home at some point even though we weren't as sure) home and knew all the residents on her floor immediately.

One thing about my grandmother was that she was an extremely kind person and tried to be as social as possible. So, she filled her days with Bingo, crafts, and talking to other residents. I often pushed her through the halls and she pointed out each person and shared their story.

Two years was the amount of time she was a resident at the nursing facility. A doctor new to her team deemed her able to live on her own even though she was still wheelchair bound and we moved her home.

Two weeks later, my dad called my mom's house at 1:00 in afternoon. I was home. I think had a half day of school that day and my dad should have been at work. It was extremely unusual for him to call my mom's house at all, let alone during the middle of his work day and ask if my mom was home. My parents didn't hate each other, but they were divorced for a reason and avoided contact with each other when possible.

My dad didn't give me any information over the phone. He simply told me to have my mom call him when she got home. As soon as I hung up the phone, I immediately knew something was wrong. Even though my grandmother returned home, her health was still concerning.

I knew no one would answer before I dialed, but I carefully pressed the numbers of her line into the cordless phone in the kitchen. Since this was 1996, cell phones were not popular, and everyone still had landlines. I called my grandmother every single day since she came home. However, I missed two days. I didn't call the last two days. Not for any particular reason, but just because in my mind, I thought she heard enough of me, and my mind was at ease just enough to not smother her with attention.

I let my guard down and thought she was going to be ok. When her voice was not at the other end, I knew. She was gone. It took until the evening to officially hear the news. My mom took me over to my dad's house 15 minutes away and they sat me down on the camel-colored sectional sofa that my parents owned before I was born. The look in their eyes said everything, so I initiated the conversation. I said, "something happened to Grammy" and they nodded. I think I asked if she was dead and there was another nod.

Instead of crying, I sat there like a stone, unmovable and unreadable. I can't remember what I did or said, but I remember feeling nothing, being absolutely numb. My first taste of trauma, my first close loss, my person was gone.

The reason I tell this story is because this loss occurred when I was 13, two months before my 14th birthday. Cole's first taste of trauma, his cancer diagnosis, occurred 21 days after his 14th birthday. We both experienced a traumatic event around the age of 14.

Trauma in the teenage years occurs at such a pivotal point in development and can have a large impact on one's social, emotional, mental and physical health later in life. My trauma resulted in an eating disorder that still haunts me 27 years later. This brings me to the aspect of mental health, healing and uncovering the invisible scars residing under the surface of the trauma.

I don't want other people to have these types of stories, especially teenage cancer patients. The trauma of diagnosis is enough in and of itself. It should not spur new struggles in this vulnerable population. For this reason, I am a huge advocate of social, emotional, and mental health support from diagnosis through end of treatment and beyond.

Recently, I completed a survey about the social/emotional support we had at our treating hospital and after answering all the questions I came to a startling realization. The mental health support we were offered during treatment was little to non-existent. Now, I am not writing this to point fingers at our hospital, but if my son received very little mental health support, I'm betting many other pediatric cancer patients are in the same position.

I cannot emphasize the importance of having the psychology team present from the very beginning. I firmly believe a mental health evaluation and learning assessment should be done at the beginning of treatment along with all the standard physical assessments like echocardiograms and CT scans. A baseline mental and learning assessment will give the treating team clues as to how chemo has affected the patient's learning, mental, and emotional well-being later on during the treatment journey and throughout their life.

Without a baseline assessment, we cannot measure the amount of destruction chemo may have caused and develop a plan for further support. Cancer diagnosis and treatment are scary for anyone, let alone someone in the midst of developing into an adult. Without a mental health team, we can only speculate the destruction chemo, trauma, and missing out on everyday teenage things while being poked, prodded, and filled with poison can cause.

With assessment, psychological tests and a team of professionals behind each patient from start to finish and beyond, the effects of a traumatic diagnosis and years of treatment can be measured and treated specifically instead of blindly assuming our teens were affected by their journey and not knowing the extent of such effects.

I am such an advocate for mental health support because we didn't have any. I lied. We had minimal support. When I say minimal support I mean, after I requested to have a psychologist come into the clinic room, a resident came and spoke to Cole on three different occasions (two different residents) during the beginning of his treatment.

I was in the room the entire time and they stayed maybe 15 or 20 minutes, asking baseline and surface level questions. I'm assuming this wasn't helpful because Cole never wanted them to come back after the initial visits and they were far too busy to come up to clinic regularly.

Besides asking the obligatory mental health questions during their assessment, the doctors never pushed the issue. Since the hospital had a skeleton crew in the psychology department and little to no pediatric specialists, they knew there wasn't much to offer in the way of support.

I hear about bigger support networks in larger hospitals and I want a future where this is standard no matter where a patient is treated. Mental health sessions, therapeutic play, music therapy, art therapy and learning assessments should all be incorporated into the treatment plan. Especially, when the medication used can cause significant issues later in life.

Our teens have suffered enough trauma throughout the journey to warrant a support team behind them. The invisible scars cannot be seen by the naked eye, but a mental health professional can uncover the scars and begin to treat and heal the entire person.

Physical scars are visible while emotional scars, the remnants left behind by a traumatic experience, are often invisible and the signs of emotional trauma and its effects are hard to notice if you don't know what you are looking for. An experience such as a pediatric cancer diagnosis is traumatic for not only the patient, but the entire family as well.

I want to describe a recent experience that caught me off guard. A few weeks ago, Cole was treated for strep throat because his brother tested positive and after a look in his mouth by the acute care provider, she decided there was no need for a swab. She was going to treat him for strep regardless due to his medical history, the look of his throat, and Kaden's positive swab. This may seem odd, but given Cole's medical history and presentation with his sore throat and patches resembling strep, the provider felt confident enough to order the antibiotics.

Well, a couple of days later, Cole developed a pretty nasty cough which isn't really a sign of strep and his pediatrician expressed that she wished the acute care provider would have swabbed him for strep to have the actual test results to back the treatment because they were seeing a number of cases of a virus that causes some pretty nasty looking throat symptoms. This virus was more likely the culprit due to the cough and lack of other strep related symptoms.

This was the first fever and significant illness Cole experienced after treatment and the trauma snuck up on me immediately. Sitting in that same room to get blood counts because Cole was lethargic, sent me into an immediate panic.

I texted one of my cancer mom friends that I needed her to help me calm down. I immediately received a phone call with a soft and empathetic voice on the other end. As I walked outside to take the call and relay my story to the person on the other side, a state away, I started to feel better.

I didn't feel better because the trauma had passed and someone had a magic wand to make it all disappear. I felt better because my friend, upon hearing my story, immediately divulged a very similar story she experienced the prior week. Her daughter was out of treatment for four years and she had a very similar reaction to mine with frantic phone calls asking her friends to calm her crazy after her daughter became ill with a cold. I felt seen. I felt understood. I felt a part of a group who experienced the same things.

One thing to realize about trauma is that it is extremely sneaky. Everything can seem and feel fine. Sometimes I even ask myself why I'm not reacting to something I normally would be anxious about and get nervous that I'm not experiencing anxiety.

What the heck kind of demented reasoning is that? Creating anxiety because you didn't experience anxiety. Yep, that's what we are dealing with. Trauma doesn't follow rules. It sneaks around and pops up when you least expect it.

Have you ever watched those videos on your phone or computer that seem like everything is fine and then all of a sudden, a monster, spider, or something else scary bursts onto the screen accompanied by a loud noise? I can't watch those types of videos because I will literally pee my pants. Well, trauma is like that. It wants you to pee your pants, lose your cool, and be overwhelmed by anxiety and stress.

If you have ever been incapacitated by trauma, stress, anxiety, or panic you know that it is absolutely no fun. Prior to Cole's diagnosis, I thought I had anxiety. Well, let me rephrase that…I did have diagnosed anxiety, but I had no clue how when trauma enters the picture, the level of anxiety, coupled with panic, can increase to an immeasurable level.

I still suffer from panic attacks and anxiety and probably always will. Our entire family went through something unimaginable, and I was (and still am) unable to process it on some days. I have a friend who is very into positive psychology and the science behind how our brain elicits certain responses in our body. This science has helped me to understand why I am reacting the way I am and what to do when such reactions occur.

If you like learning about the brain and the reasoning behind our responses, definitely look up some articles or books on positive psychology. It is very interesting, informative, and helpful. The calming techniques and breathing exercises that accompany this school of thought have also been very instrumental in my healing.

So, I've already discussed that trauma is sneaky, aims to scare the crap out of us, is unpredictable and causes certain responses in our body, including panic. Trauma also makes me very irritable, and I tend to yell a lot more than I did before Cole was diagnosed. It's almost as if I can't handle one thing going wrong because I am already on high alert and once it happens, I lose it. I yell, scream, jump out of my chair or respond in some other overly dramatic way. In the back of my mind, I understand my response is not normal and I also know where it originated but it is something I am working on and trying to manage.

I recognize my responses in myself and know when stress is about to rear its ugly head. My body gets tense, my breathing becomes shallow, and I feel completely overwhelmed and absent from my surroundings. Recognizing that stress is overwhelming me, I can employ a relaxation tactic like a breathing exercise or simply remove myself from the situation and go outside, surrounding myself in the light and warmth of the sun.

Finding a technique that works can be challenging. I explored many different options like running, art, taking a nap, crafting, reading, yoga, breathing, and mindfulness. Like anything, these techniques will not be beneficial unless they are practiced regularly. Focusing on one thing at a time helps me as well. It seems to be a common thread in this book.

"One day at a time"
One hour at a time
One moment at a time
One thing at a time

One anything at a time, really. Live in the moment and take things step-by-step. When I find that I am overwhelmed, it is truly because too much is happening at once. If I take it back and simplify my life, I am able to process what is happening and lessen my stress response. I used to take for granted that I had minimal stress, and I didn't need these techniques to function on a daily basis. Well, I also did not walk my child through a cancer journey at that point, so it makes sense that the stress was significantly lower in the absence of trauma.

Give yourself grace, seek what you need, fight for what your child needs to support their mental health, and take it "one day at a time".

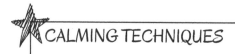

Box Breathing

Get into a comfortable and safe sitting position and close your eyes if you wish. Imagine a box or square and trace the imaginary box on your arm, leg, or object near you. As you go up the one side, breathe in for five seconds. When you get to the corner, hold your breath for five seconds. When you go across the top, let your breath out for the count of five. When you reach the corner, hold for five and continue the pattern. Trace the box. Breathe in for five. Hold for five. Breathe out for five. Hold for five. Breath in for five, etc. Breathing in at the imaginary sides of the box, holding at the imaginary corners, you will feel relaxed, almost as if you just completed a workout and your muscles and body are relaxed and calm. You can start at any count if five is too much to begin. As you practice, you can lengthen the counts.

Mindfulness

The technique I described above is a type of mindfulness. There are many other techniques that focus on the present when managing anxiety and stress.

Many different schools of thought and differing practices exist within the mindfulness realm. The basics all revolve around:

Living in the present- pay attention to everything around you and slow yourself down taking everything in.

Engaging the senses (the 5-4-3-2-1 exercise below is a great example)

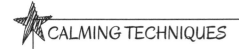# CALMING TECHNIQUES

Accepting yourself in that moment in time without judgement

Breathwork- many practices involve breathing and meditation

The body scan is one activity that helped me on occasion. I have a difficult time with meditation of any kind. It takes practice. If done regularly there are great benefits. YouTube is a great resource for body scan tutorials.

<u>Exercise</u>
Walking, workouts, swimming, running, tennis, the options are endless. Exercise and physical activity done regularly has great mental health benefits, lessening the symptoms of depression and anxiety.

<u>5-4-3-2-1 Technique</u>
By focusing on the present moment and engaging the sense allowing the calm to take over the anxiousness. In this technique you find:

5 Things you can see-
Describe (in your head or out loud) five things that you see at that moment

4 Things you can touch-
Touch or hold four things that are close to you

CALMING TECHNIQUES

3 things you can hear-
Identify three sounds

2 things you can smell-
Identify 2 smells

1 thing you can taste-
I usually put a piece of gum, a mint, or candy in my mouth at this point.

Resources and supplies
I am a huge advocate for fidget toys and items. Giving your hands something to do and focus on helps calm your brain. Great for anxiety, ADHD, stress, and general unrest, sensory issues.

Some of my favorites are:
Putty- moldable, stretchable

Push bubble bracelets

Tangles

Spiky Rings

Box Breath Stickers

There is a company (probably more than one) than makes textured stickers you can place on the back of your phone or other convenient place to trace as you practice your box breathing.

CHAPTER 11

Never Forget, Always Advocate and
Spread Awareness Like Confetti

From the moment of diagnosis, I went into this journey with the mindset "if I can help make it even just a little bit easier for someone going through the fight" I will find my purpose.

Laura

From day one of this experience, I always had the mindset that our family had no choice about whether or not we were going on this journey. It's never a choice. If another family has to go through this arduous and unforgiving journey, I will do what I can to make it just a bit easier for them than it was for us. I will never waste the knowledge, experiences, and connections we made over the last three years.

Having that goal in mind, when the trauma dissipated and the dust settled in my brain, allowing the capacity to take on supporting others, I dove in. Every opportunity that presented itself was an opportunity to spread awareness, support another mother or caregiver, and ease some of the pain that is childhood cancer.

I often replay and overanalyze my life experiences, questioning what I could do next time or how I could help someone else going through something similar. I don't do it for recognition. Actually, being in the spotlight is one of the things that holds me back from doing more. I don't mind opening up to others and I'm not intimidated by public speaking. I can usually advocate without any problems, however there are times when it hits me all at once. The anxiety and lasting effects of the trauma are too much and I shut down. I realized this early in my advocacy and have learned to say no and be selective in the opportunities I pursue.

I wish I could do everything and I'm sure other advocates feel the same way. However, saying "yes" to every opportunity I am presented is humanely impossible. Learning to say "no" and prioritizing my advocacy experiences has definitely become a necessary approach even though it's difficult at times.

While Cole was still in treatment and experiencing a drug shortage of Erwinase®, I knew other families would be affected by the limited supply of this life-saving poison. What an oxymoron, right? Once we secured Cole's doses, the only thing on my mind was making sure the other patients who needed this drug got it and got it on time.

Due to the size of our hospital, at the time, there was only one other patient who needed Erwinase®. The patient reacted while we were in the middle of our search for the drug, so the doctors and nurses approached me because they knew I was working with *Angels for Change* and anticipated this patient needing the drug that was nowhere to be found.

Since we couldn't find any vials for Cole and were searching day and night, we knew it was going to be nearly impossible to find it for someone else too.

Luckily there was a trial drug in the last phases of being tested and since this patient didn't yet receive any doses of Erwinase®, they would qualify for the trial if we could get them into a nearby hospital. Keeping this patient's story anonymous and allowing them privacy, I will not divulge their story. What I will share, however, is because I worked together with Laura Bray and advocated for another patient things worked out favorably.

I was so grateful that the hospital team, *Angels for Change*, and the patient and their family trusted me and looked to me for guidance in solving this issue. Drug shortages are not an easy situation for anyone, the hospital included. I was honored to use my knowledge and connections to help someone else, hopefully making the experience easier for them than it was for us.

The patient received all doses of this medicine on time and the drug passed the trial and is officially a replacement drug for Erwinase®. Due to the amazing advocacy of Laura Bray and *Angels for Change*, many other families will get to say they received their medication on time and will not have to worry about a shortage of RYLAZE® (the trial drug which is now an approved alternate drug for PEG-asparaginase) for the foreseeable future.

Besides helping families navigate drug shortages, I was also lucky enough to be asked several times to connect with newly diagnosed families who didn't know where to turn. Since COVID was in full swing, human interaction was very limited. Our amazing social worker was determined to give the families the support they so desperately craved by connecting families with similar diagnoses.

One of the families I was able to connect with ended up supporting me as well. In the beginning I gave them information, support, and a shoulder to cry on. Throughout treatment, the mom of the fighter was there for me more than once. Knowing I was sought out to give support to other patients simply because of our experience and in turn these families were also there for us every step of the way, creates a bond like no other.

Sure, if COVID was nonexistent, there would have been many more options for connection, but we did what we could with what we were dealt, and it does not diminish the experience to any extent.

In a perfect world, I imagine families gathered inpatient sharing a meal together. I can also see families gathered downstairs at the fountain which lies in the lobby, a peaceful area where the sound of water trickling down the green porous surface of the frog in the middle of a mosaic blue tile pool of clear, cool water fills the area. Families are socializing, drinking coffee, and enjoying the atmosphere outside of the stark and solemn hospital room.

I hope that after COVID many of these things can resume, including families gathering in the hallways with their warriors attached to IV poles pumping poison in their veins, to take a stroll together in solidarity, knowing the struggles that happen behind all the closed hospital room doors. Leaving the room and interacting with another patient and their caregiver refuels both you and your warrior.

Support groups, in person and online, were another goal of mine. I tried so hard to bring a group to our hospital, but it wasn't the right time. We tried month after month and rarely had a participant. I didn't mind taking the hour and sitting on my computer interacting with hospital staff and our group facilitator but at some point, I couldn't keep putting in the effort when other things were begging for my time and attention.

Eventually, the decision was made to put the group on hold and hopefully someday another parent will take hold and bring this amazing group to life, supporting other caregivers in the fight.

Another good thing that came from my connections was the ability to connect Momcology® to our hospital. My hopes are that in connecting a well-known caregiver support organization to our caregivers, they will be able to seek the support they need and know the resource exists. I found out about this group through another cancer mom whose child was treated at a much larger hospital. The organization had a support group right in the hospital which was amazing. Now the social workers and child life specialists regularly share the Momcology® information with caregivers at our hospital. Caregivers now have the knowledge of an amazing group with thousands of cancer moms around the country, willing and ready to support at a moment's notice.

One common thread in childhood cancer parents and caregivers is the willingness to drop everything and be there for another family because we have been there and know firsthand how awful it can be and how alone you can feel. I never want anyone to feel alone in the journey.

There are so many ways I wish I could help other families, but I need to realize I am doing what I can and if I make it easier for just one more family, I will meet my goal. Due to our harrowing experience and trauma week upon week, I will never stop advocating for others. I know, firsthand, how horrible pediatric cancer is. This is something I could not say three years ago. I was naïve and blind to this terrible disease, and it was ignorant bliss.

I didn't know how children were dying because they couldn't get the medicine necessary to save their lives. Here in America, the land of plenty, it was unheard of to not be able to get your medication, right? That only happened in Third World countries or areas too poor to vaccinate their children or provide medication to the sick. No, it happens every single day right in your town or city. Not only did it happen to my son, but it also happened to my father a few months later.

It's not fair that a person fighting for their life can't get a medication that is made to save them. The tools need to be available for the protocol to work. This is not solely a pediatric cancer issue. Many types of medication land themselves on the National Drug Shortage list due to manufacturing and supply chain issues. Priority needs to be placed on making any type of life-saving medication readily available, accessible, and affordable to all patients in need.

Because Cole experienced a drug shortage during treatment, I am very aware of the effects of not obtaining medication on time. Due to the delay of a course of chemo, a life-threatening diabetic reaction occurred in my child causing him to need insulin each subsequent time the medication was administered.

Our patients go through enough at such a young age. Worrying about receiving the medicine they so desperately need on time should not be a worry placed upon their souls. Due to enduring such a hardship, every time I hear of another medication on the shortage list or another patient desperately trying to find medication, my heart is on fire and my soul longs to help.

Undergoing a pediatric cancer journey is the hardest thing our family has gone through, by far. The fire that burns for other families going through a similar journey will never smolder, it will always be there in our hearts. Therefore, I will always help. Even though it rips my heart apart each time I hear of another family going through a diagnosis, a warrior becoming an angel, or a child having a side effect from chemo, I have the mindset that if someone is experiencing something in which I can help, I will. Since we had no choice and were chosen to endure this battle, anything and everything I can do to support my family and other families is all I can do.

You may notice Cole did not write a section on this chapter. I feel it is necessary to explain why some chapters may not have a "Cole" section. From the beginning of our writing journey, I gave Cole a choice in every aspect of the book and the public events that follow. Advocacy and a burning desire to help others is my passion. So, I had a lot to say on the subject. Cole certainly has the same desire, but he is more laid back and behind the scenes in his approach.

It's extremely important to me to always give Cole a choice because for over three years, his ability to choose in many aspects of his life was non-existent.

CHAPTER 12

Scars

"Out of suffering have emerged the strongest souls; the most massive characters are seared with scars." - Khalil Gibran

Laura

As we navigate life, we live through experiences. Some are positive, some negative, and many are impactful in one way or another. Some of these experiences are so significant because after we experience them, our life fills two distinct categories: before the event and after the event. How we continue to live life in the "after" is solely dependent upon the experience itself and the lasting impact on one's life. These abstract experiences I am talking about fit in many categories like trauma in general, an accident, a huge milestone, a large accomplishment, or even winning the lottery.

However, for the purpose of this book, I'm talking about a cancer diagnosis. If you or someone close to you experiences a cancer diagnosis, life takes on a very different meaning. Time is now put into two very distinct buckets. The before diagnosis bucket and the now bucket.

When I think about the "before bucket," I imagine a bright, shiny, and new vessel. Maybe it is colorful or has a pretty design painted upon its surface. The bucket is in great condition and looks as if it could be sitting on a store shelf, unused. I use this perfect bucket to represent what life was like before our pediatric cancer diagnosis. So, in my specific experience, I'm referencing any day before January 15, 2020.

Although the bucket may look perfect when looking back in time and remembering life experiences in the before category, the truth is life was still difficult. However, the pre-cancer difficultly level is nowhere near the difficulty level of now. Negative experiences still occurred, but now that we have experienced the mother of all negative experiences, the kids not getting up for school, driving two hours each way to a hockey game, or a dog who won't pee outside are considered minor inconveniences and life is appreciated on a whole new dimension when something so volatile as cancer threatens to take it all away. The "big" things in our before are now little nuisances in our after and not worth the fight.

Now when we imagine the after bucket, I'm sure you can guess it doesn't look like the before bucket at all. The weathered, dirty, beaten down, full of holes and rusted bucket whose rose-colored design is now foggy and un-viewable is full of hard experiences and tough life decisions. This bucket has been through a lot. Cancer takes that beautiful before bucket containing everything that was once easy and beats it down, making it weary from battle. Even in our current state of after treatment, the damage to the bucket is so severe that the markings and weathered nature are hard to ignore. Over time, the holes are patched, the design redrawn, and dirt washed off, but the trauma is still noticeable and nothing looks as it did before.

Along with the look of our battle-worn bucket, we also developed some scars along the way. No one goes through life unscathed, though the number, nature, and look of everyone's scars differ. Scars are physical marks on our bodies as opposed to a whole separate vessel like a bucket that we carry with us. The bucket can be put down and returned to at another time, but scars, they never leave us. The scars of cancer are not always physical. They are often emotional, mental, social, and invisible.

Scars not seen are often the most painful and misunderstood. Visible scars show others a story regarding a battle which left its mark upon the body of the warrior. Using the clues visible scars give us to make assumptions about the type of battle is like a guide to another language or a cipher of illness and struggle. Physical manifestations differ widely. While some battle marks can be small, large, thick, thin, painful, bumpy, hard to see or very visible, the invisible scars are a phantom code impossible to break. Depending on the location, physical scars can be hidden but often, the scars are in full view of others to scrutinize, wonder, or ask questions regarding the marks on our bodies we carry everywhere.

Scars are reminders of walking through a difficult experience and surviving. As I type, I'm looking down at my left wrist at the scar running from the base of my hand about three inches up my arm. Almost exactly one year to the day I am typing these words, I underwent surgery for a badly broken wrist. The experience of breaking myself and being the center of medical attention after we had been through so much with Cole the past three years was anxiety provoking. I was so used to having my attention on Cole and his medical condition that undergoing an injury myself pushed me over the edge.

Even though we had been on this journey for almost three years at that point, Cole was still in treatment and in the maintenance phase. So, we tried to do things as a family and get Cole out a little more than the prior two years. From about age four to age ten, Cole played ice hockey as did his brother. He was amazing to watch on the ice. It looked as if he were dancing on the surface of the ice and carefully guiding the puck where he needed it to go. The skating looked effortless as did the puck handling and stickwork. It wasn't uncommon for Cole to score a hattrick or three goals during one game.

We still tried to get to the rink often to skate. Due to Cole's diagnosis and COVID, it was almost two years since our last visit. February 13, 2022 was the day we finally got back on the ice. I remember this date well because it's also the day I so gracefully fell while gliding along the ice. I wasn't doing anything fancy and I was even holding my husband's hand at the time. I also attempted to break my fall by outstretching my arm. Not a good idea. I understand it was a reflex, but it also caused my wrist to break. I later told everyone at the hospital I tripped while doing a Triple Lutz, which is an extremely graceful looking jump. Everyone laughed at my story, except for one grumpy nurse in the ER triage.

When I am in pain, physically or mentally, I use humor as a way to lighten the mood. Another joke I told was my affinity for winter sports and injuries, explaining the only two broken bones I had during my almost 40 years of life, were while competing in some type of winter sport. This was more of a funny story than a joke because it was entirely true. My first broken wrist occurred while snowboarding (on the bunny slope) on the one and only day my mom ever let me skip school.

So, I wasn't brand new to how a broken bone felt but wow, this was way worse. I knew immediately when I tried to get up and I couldn't move my wrist or hold up my arm. I looked like an injured seal, unable to scurry off the ice, its flipper bent and hanging in an awkward way. What is even better is my pain response. Everyone reacts to pain differently and each situation can differ. I usually have a pretty good threshold for pain, but for some reason, I started crying uncontrollably for hours until my arm was numbed, and the bones set back into place.

I'll never forget the lady who kept staring at me as my husband gently guided me off the ice, supporting and cradling me like an egg out of its carton, unprotected and vulnerable. Literally, the lady wasn't even on the ice. She was standing right outside the rink walls and peering at me through the glass like I was an injured fish in an aquarium.

I did give her a mean girl look and almost told her to stop staring. Obviously, not my finest moment and I was in a ton of pain so the last thing I wanted was someone staring at me while I bawled my eyes out from the amount of pain my lack of grace caused. She was probably thinking I was a huge baby. Well, guess what lady? I had a Colles fracture, a fracture of the distal radius bone of the forearm seen widely in the elderly. So, there.

I had a painful fracture followed by surgery and a weird scar to prove my story. Oh, and I also have a plate in my arm so I'm sure I'll be fun going through the metal detectors from now on.

Anyway, the above story gives me a few lessons. Don't stare. It's not nice. Also, people respond differently to each situation so give grace and don't be mean. I'm glad I only gave her a dirty look and didn't yell. I would have felt awful.

Another lesson I get is from my scar itself. When I look down at my wrist, I think about the difficult injury I experienced and everything I went through for about four months. I also think, "four months". I had it difficult for four months. Cole had treatment for almost three years and more than one scar to prove it.

Let's take a rundown of some of the traumatic experiences Cole endured...

Scar #1: the undeniable port scar. Being a cancer family, I am able to recognize the port scar on an individual a mile away. It's a battle wound and mark of a soldier. Cole's is kind of weird and very visible for a couple of reasons. The first reason is that his first port became infected right after placement. He only had it about five weeks, if that, and the incision never healed because the port was located directly under the incision.

So, when the nurses accessed it over and over again the incision was disturbed and grew a weird pink tissue infection. There are several reasons that may explain why Cole's first port never healed and include the port placement directly under his scar, the massive number of steroid doses he was prescribed during the induction phase, or the amount of fluid he was on in the hospital causing a shift to the port after his body expelled the fluid and became less marshmallow man puffy. Whatever the reason, it definitely became infected, and his amazing team noticed it right away, scheduling removal that same day.

The port was removed and a new port was placed six weeks later in the same spot. So, when the area finally healed, Cole's scar developed a keloid which is a fancy name for a pronounced, bumpy, scar. We were told some people just make good scars and some skin is more likely to develop a keloid. Our story regarding Cole's port serves to show things happen for a reason. From day one, there were issues with the port. As soon as the new port was placed, we never had port issues again. Almost three years after placement, it still worked like a charm and accessing the device was easy-peasy and caused minimal discomfort.

Scar #2 has to do with the port as well and is a small little "nick" by Cole's collarbone. This scar occurred when a tiny incision was made to guide the wire of the port to his aorta. It's a tiny scar and chances are, the scar itself may not be visible in a few years. The tiny scar is part of a huge event. Even though it's small, the scar is partnered with the big port scar and the insertion and removal of the device responsible for delivering the poison through his veins and throughout his bloodstream quicker than if given via IV in the arm. The port also made fevers really fun for our family because anytime Cole spiked a fever higher than a certain degree, we were off to the hospital and admitted. The little scar also indicated the placement of a port which meant there were two big things Cole could not do which were swimming in public pools, lakes, creeks, ponds, or anywhere that wasn't extremely well cared for and chlorinated, and participate in any type of contact sport. So, even though little "nick" was small and may not be visible in the future, it is part of a bigger and more serious event.

Scar #3 is hardly visible thanks to an amazing surgeon and is located in

Cole's belly button. Funny story, Cole had a messed-up belly button to begin his life. When he was born at 36 weeks, the doctors and nurses present in the delivery room numbered at least 8-10 and, I'm not going to lie, made me panic a bit. Because he was a little early, they wanted to make sure everything was ok and tend to anything that was concerning, immediately. In their haste, one of the team clipped his skin in the umbilical clip leaving a wonky looking belly button resembling two little tiny butt cheeks. He is going to be so mad at me.

Anyway, his belly button was always weird. So, when he had a ruptured appendix, the surgeon went through his belly button leaving a little line and unrecognizable button of any kind. He did an amazing job. What should have been Cole's largest scar by far signifying an experience that could have killed my son, is one of the least noticeable. The ruptured appendix and subsequent surgery and hospital stay were definitely a trying time as was the news that his appendix was positive for EBV, but it's the scar that is healed and hidden due to the amazing experience and knowledge of a capable surgeon and great medical team.

Even though the physical scar is barely able to be seen, the invisible scar was great. Cole was in extreme pain for weeks and struggled greatly to stand, move around, eat, and be active. It took months for him to get back to being himself. The anxiety and depression caused by this experience cannot be measured but it was noticed by our family, medical team, and friends. I cannot begin to imagine the experience of being ripped away from normal life once again to endure a traumatic surgery, week-long hospital admission, and painful recovery just as things returned to our kind of normal and Cole was at the one-year mark left of treatment.

We didn't know this at the time, but this harrowing experience is responsible for the end of treatment on October 3, 2022 instead of May 23, 2023 which was the original end of treatment date.

Sometimes, scars indicate experiences working out for the better and a strange turn of events only explainable by God's hands moving all the pieces together to create the best scenario for Cole and allow all his scars to heal and become reminders of the strength, endurance, and bravery he exhibits every single day.

Cole

I have a few scars from my cancer journey that will be with me throughout my life. The biggest and most noticeable scar is my port scar that marks me as a survivor. Since getting my port placed and going through treatment, I've noticed the same scar on others. I know exactly what they have been through because I have walked a similar path.

The scars throughout my body are reminders of my journey and how far I have come in the last three years. I have been through many different experiences, a lot of them involving pain both physical and mental. I told myself that I needed to push through and keep going. The scars signify accomplishments throughout my treatment.

The port being placed meant treatment could start and when the scar healed, it meant I was even further into treatment and one thing was checked off the list of my journey. The same scar at the end of treatment had a very different meaning. There was no longer a port just under my skin. The port was gone as it was not needed anymore. I was now a survivor.

One of my other scars marks a really hard time during treatment. When my appendix ruptured, it was one of the most painful experiences in my life and an even harder recovery. The scar really isn't noticeable, but I know it's there. When I look down at my stomach, I remember the pain and the difficult recovery. When I look at myself today I can see how far I've come and all the things I had to push through to get to this place.

Right after surgery, I couldn't really walk far or stand for long. It hurt to sit and get out of the bed, so my mom bought me a wedge type pillow to prevent me from lying flat. Since I laid at an angle, it was a little easier to get to a sitting position and then stand. I was so weak I could not stand or walk for more than a few moments. I also remember how nauseous I was for a few days after the surgery and how scared I was to throw up. It was so painful. I can't believe I went from not even being able to stand to getting ready for my senior football season. I can work out at the gym, lift weights, and do workouts with the team. I feel mostly back to normal and continue to push each day to get stronger and faster. When I look at my stomach, I see the mark of a warrior.

The port scar reminds me of my entire journey and all the battles I faced while the appendectomy scar signifies an extremely hard battle as a result of treatment. This side effect ultimately led to the hospitals' decision to end treatment and open the port scar once again to remove the device that gave me treatment for over three long years.

The scars that hurt the most are those that cannot be seen. Cancer is horrible and a really hard journey. Going through this journey while being a teenager was really difficult. All the things I experienced over the past couple of years were things that no one should have to go through, let alone as a child or teen. In addition to the physical pain that cancer causes and the actual marks on my body that remind me of the pain and sickness, there is the emotional pain and anxiety that cancer leaves behind.

I always had anxiety to some extent. Sometimes it is worse than others and even though I am out of treatment, the cancer left anxiety and depression behind as scars. I have to keep reminding myself that I am a survivor. I went through years of a traumatic journey, and I didn't do it alone. That means I don't have to do it alone now.

Since these scars are invisible no one can see or know they exist. For those teens going through a diagnosis right now or survivors who finished their battle, remember if there are hard days or more battles in your head, reach out and get your team behind you once again. Take each battle you face, whether it is physical or mental, one at a time. If you need a reminder of your strength and bravery, take a look at your scars and remember how far you have come.

"Never be ashamed of a scar. It simply means you were stronger than whatever tried to hurt you." – Unknown

"The one that has the most scar's wins the game life offers us". – Paul Reichert

CHAPTER 13

Siblings

Superheroes standing near the sidelines watching and waiting to be tagged into the fight. Pediatric cancer siblings, our fighters' biggest heroes and supporters but they need support, too!

Laura

When I was four years old, my parents separated and continued to live separate lives until their divorce was finalized when I was seven. My parents were married for 10 years before I was born, but soon realized their problems weren't solved by having a child and decided to part ways. Therefore, I never had the opportunity to have a sibling. I grew up alone in two very different houses. I had an amazing childhood, with very loving parents, but always wondered what it would be like to not be alone.

Sure, I had friends and cousins, but I didn't live with anyone who was near my age and never had the bond of a sibling. Therefore, I always knew I wanted more than one child and I wanted them to be close in age so they could grow up together, always having each other to turn to whenever they needed.

When Cole was 18 months old, we found out my dream was going to come true. I was pregnant with our second child. We were completely overjoyed, and I felt a sense of calm knowing Cole was not going to grow up alone and he would have a sibling.

Little did I know that Cole and Kaden would be complete opposites in every sense of the word. Starting with the pregnancies.

Cole was four weeks early, had his days and nights mixed up, and was extremely colicky. Kaden was almost late (I had the option of an induction five days before his due date and took it with no second guessing), slept through the night by four months old and was a pretty easy baby. Cole was always my more difficult child when he was younger and Kaden was pretty easy going until he was about six years old.

The tables then turned, and Kaden was cranky, difficult, and rebellious while Cole was now easy going. My two perfect boys are never on the same page. When one is cranky, the other is happy and when one is content the other is jumping off the walls. Cole is athletic and has an easy time in school, getting stellar grades. Kaden has dyslexia and dysgraphia (trouble with writing) and the attention span of my German Shepherd, Bo. School has always been difficult for Kaden as he learns differently than the general population. He loves to ride dirt bikes, be outside and work with his hands.

The above description of my children's characteristics is mentioned for a reason. My perfect little sibling team in my mind is not reality. My kids never got along super well. I chalk it up to the fact that they are not similar in any way shape or form. Actually, they are completely opposite. Now, they don't hate each other or run in the opposite direction when one approaches, but their relationship is not typical. Never having had a sibling, I realize there may not be a typical sibling relationship and everything in our family may be totally normal. The more I think about it, I'm sure it was just the fantasy in my mind that gave me the delusion of a TV perfect sibling team.

One characteristic I failed to mention is their overall personalities. Kaden loves big and publicly. You absolutely know he loves you because he hugs, kisses, smothers, and tells you constantly. Cole is super reserved and doesn't often mention his feelings. He bottles everything up and places it in a deep, dark corner. Never really knowing where you stand with Cole, I have come to understand this child is exactly how I was before becoming a mom. I was pretty reserved, quiet, and emotionless. So, when Kaden comes at Cole with a full-force epic hulk hug and smothering "I love you", it's easy to see Cole's reaction. What else do boys do except for epic WWE wrestling moves when comforted with affection?

Sibling relationships were always just in my mind. Having never experienced the love of a sibling myself, it's easy to see how my perfect sibling love was flawed. Only ever having seen these types of relationships on TV, it's easy to see how I wasn't exactly accurate. Even though their relationship isn't what I envisioned a sibling relationship consisting of, it is perfect. They love in their own way, and they will always be each other's best friend and safe haven throughout their lives.

When Cole was diagnosed, Kaden was immediately displaced. All focus was on our oldest son and saving his life. The moment I received the call telling me that Cole had leukemia, the only thing I could focus upon was how to cure him, doing whatever it takes. I immediately scooped up Cole and took him to the ER as I was instructed. My husband stayed home with Kaden until my parents could come to watch him as it was the evening and we didn't know how long we would be gone. Kaden was only 11 at the time, far too young to be left to himself.

Though, my stepdad was there to take Kaden to my parents' home and be with him while my husband, my mom, my cousin, and I were surrounding Cole with prayers at the hospital, we did leave Kaden alone. All of us completely focused on Cole and his dire condition at the time and we had no room for any other thoughts. In the meantime, Kaden was expected to continue his life while his brother was in the hospital fighting to live. Staying with his grandparents, going to school, and continuing with most of his day-to-day activities while everything was turned upside down, was the reality of my 11-year-old and many other pediatric cancer siblings.

Even though we made sure Kaden was taken care of, we did leave him. When everything was extremely confusing and traumatic, he was expected to continue on in his life like nothing had changed. Everything was now different, and he was living in two houses much like I did throughout my childhood. However, there was the element of uncertainty and the omnipresent worry and trauma regarding his brother's cancer diagnosis.

Pediatric cancer siblings are expected to continue on as if nothing happened when in reality, everything is a mess and nothing is the same. Most resources are focused on pediatric cancer patients with little left for the siblings. Making sure Kaden was included and felt supported was always a priority for us. During Cole's treatment, we tried to be as upfront about things as we could and we also tried to have at least one of us stay at home with Kaden while the other was with Cole. Dividing ourselves for our children helped to give some sort of normalcy to Kaden in a very un-normal time. No blueprint or guide exists for how to support a pediatric cancer sibling or a way to minimize the trauma and after effects of such a journey.

I really can't be sure how this experience will impact any of our lives but my focus is always on minimizing its effects on my children. Both of my children were impacted by Cole's diagnosis. Our entire family felt the trauma. When I look back on some of the experiences Kaden went through and try to imagine being in his shoes as an 11-year-old, I can't even begin to think about the fear that ran through his adolescent mind.

When my mind wanders and I start to feel guilty or have thoughts that I neglected Kaden, I return my mind to the traumatic event itself and how it impacted our entire family. We did exactly what we needed to do to ensure our son had the best treatment. We also did everything in our power to make sure our other son was in good hands and being taken care of in the best possible way. Even though it was impossible for us to physically be with Kaden we knew my parents and my brother-in-law were two amazing options who made sure Kaden was supported during our hardship.

Letting guilt take over our minds does not change the situation. We did the best we could with what we were dealt. There are many things in life that we have no control over and Cole getting sick was one of those things. At that moment, Cole and his health were the priority which unfortunately distanced us from Kaden.

I'll never forget Cole's first hospital admission after his initial diagnosis. It was March 28, 2020 and the world had just shut down. We were admitted due to a fever and extremely low blood pressure (which we now believe was a reaction to PEG-asparaginase). I was alone with Cole, and Josh stayed with Kaden, because we felt so bad for leaving him with family just a little over two months prior. We were hospitalized for five or six days and it was an extremely difficult admission, partly due to COVID protocols, but also due to the fact that Kaden's birthday is April 1st.

Yep, we didn't get discharged until April 3rd and I missed my child's 12th birthday. I felt so guilty and tried to do anything possible from the hospital to make sure he had a great day. Thankfully, Josh was home with him and my mom baked Kaden an amazing chocolate cake with peanut butter icing, his favorite.

I was extremely surprised when we were discharged on the 3rd and the cake and all Kaden's presents were still in the kitchen, untouched. Immediately, the tears started to fall and this was prior to Kaden explaining that he couldn't celebrate his birthday without his brother. So, he wasn't going to eat his cake or open gifts until Cole came home. Wow, the tears started to roll.

Kaden is an amazingly kind and considerate human being. The importance of having his brother there with him for his birthday emphasized in my mind that I do have the perfect little sibling duo, my boys are amazingly supportive to each other.

Needless to say, after the not so stellar hospital food the previous five or so days, we dug right into the cake after singing *Happy Birthday*, of course.

I could continue on for pages and pages on what we did to help Kaden and tell you multiple stories of my youngest son's kindness towards his brother but this is a chapter best explained by Kaden himself. So, I devised a few questions for Kaden to provide an understanding of what someone may be going through when faced with their sibling's cancer diagnosis.

How did you feel when you heard your brother had leukemia?

I felt terrible when I heard the news. I didn't really know much about leukemia but I knew it was cancer because that was what my parents told me. No one in our family ever had cancer, but I knew it was really serious and he was really sick. I was afraid he was going to die.

When I thought of cancer before Cole got sick, I thought of really sick and dying people, and I was scared because I didn't want Cole to get sick. He was my brother and he was supposed to be there for me. I was very confused as to why Cole got cancer and I didn't. I really didn't understand why it was happening to him and not me too. I had a lot of fear in the beginning and still do sometimes that I will get cancer too. If a healthy kid like Cole who works out, eats healthy, and plays sports got cancer, it could happen to me.

Right after he was diagnosed I had the most fear that I would get sick too. Now, I realize it's not likely and my fear isn't as bad anymore.

What was it like having to go to school when Cole was in the hospital?

It was really hard to go to school while my brother was so sick. In the beginning, I didn't want to go. I was really worried about Cole and I just wanted to be with my family. I wanted my parents to explain things and I wanted to visit with Cole in the hospital.

I went to the hospital twice when he was first diagnosed, but I couldn't go again because COVID started and kids couldn't visit at that point. What made things more difficult is that I couldn't even be at home. I had to go stay with my Nanny and PapPaw. I love them and like spending time with them, but when things were so scary, I just wanted to be home with my family. I had to get up earlier and get ready for school because they lived almost a half hour away.

Also, a lot of kids at school were very mean and said horrible things to me about my brother and his diagnosis. I couldn't concentrate on anything and all I did was worry. I didn't want to be there at all I just wanted to be with my brother and my parents. When Cole came home from the hospital, it was a little easier because I was home with my parents, but it was still very hard at school. We both went to the same middle school and not having Cole there made it seem scary. I was glad when COVID sent us home because then I could be with my family all the time.

What was the biggest worry you had during that time?

I was terrified my brother was going to die.

How did you feel when Cole got support and packages in the mail?

I was jealous because I didn't get any support and he was getting things every day. Since I was 11 when he was diagnosed, I didn't understand anything about treatment or how hard it was for Cole. All I saw was that he was out of school and spent a lot of time in the hospital. He got a ton of attention and gifts.

Did any of the programs help you understand?

Not really. All I got was a letter every once in a while. There was nothing explaining the things I was dealing with or any type of support. I never met any other siblings and because of COVID, I didn't get the opportunity to go to camp with Cole in the summer.

How do you wish you were supported?

I wish there was a group of siblings that could get together and I could meet other kids whose brothers or sisters have cancer. I believe it would really help to be able to talk to someone else going through the same thing I went through so I don't feel so alone.

More programs that include siblings would help also. I understand it's very difficult for all the programs to include siblings because some cancer patients may have many siblings but if we knew of a few groups that made sure siblings were included as well it would help so they don't feel so left out.

What can we do differently so that siblings are supported too?

Involve them more in treatment. I know Cole had a child life specialist who did a lot of activities and things with him. So, if there was a group that had someone similar to a child life specialist to do crafts, art projects, group events, and other activities that would really help distract siblings and make sure they were supported and never felt like they were the only person going through something terrible like their sibling's cancer.

How did it feel to see your brother sick?

It made me very upset and I felt helpless. I wanted to do anything I could to make him feel better, but it seemed like nothing I did helped. When Cole was really sick and throwing up, I got him water or throw up bags. I always asked him if he needed anything. He was hungry for different foods a lot and I love to cook. So, I always asked him what he wanted to eat and made him anything he wanted. I still like to cook and since Cole is trying to get strong for football, I make him a lot of steak. He always tells me that my steak is the best he has ever had and that makes me feel awesome.

I made Cole a sculpture, a few paintings, cards, pictures, and wrote him notes. I always tried to do something little because I couldn't just sit there and watch him be sick. It really made me upset to see him so sick from the chemo and in pain. So, any little thing that I could do made me feel like I was at least helping in my own way.

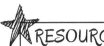 # RESOURCES FOR SIBLINGS

Alex's Lemonade Stand- Super Sibling Club

Project Outrun- Sibling Shoe Program

CHAPTER 14

After Treatment

The bell rang, signaling the end of a task. The treatment is done and the task in complete so we move onto the next phase in the journey.

Laura

Yay! You did it! It's all over, right? I wish I could tell you yes, that it's all over and everything is now behind you like looking in the rear-view mirror as you drive down the road and the farther you go the farther away the pain and trauma. But the truth is, it's not over and the trauma, anxiety, pain, and heartbreak don't magically go away at the ring of the bell.

I don't know how long it lasts or what eases the pain, but I do know that I continue to struggle. I had a particularly difficult time right after treatment for several reasons. The first reason is fear. Fear of the cancer returning and having to do this all over again. Even as I type those words, I am shuttering and my hands are shaking. The fear never goes away, and I hope with time that it gets easier, but I do know parents further out of treatment than us and they still experience this fear.

In addition to the fear is the wait. The waiting is the hardest part, right? You got it, Tom Petty. The wait followed us throughout almost every experience in this journey. There was the wait for counts, the wait for answers, the wait in the waiting room, the wait for chemo, the wait for counts to recover... I could go on and on about all the instances when we needed to wait.

After treatment, one of the hardest waits is the wait for calm. Every time Cole gets counts or has an appointment, I become extremely irritable and anxiety ridden about two days before the event. The wait is terrible. There are no immediate answers and I guess that is part of the calm in the storm. The after-treatment life. Things are going well but no I can't be happy. I am always on the lookout for anything to go wrong. I am constantly waiting for something to happen and constantly waiting for someone to calm my fears.

I feel like a person walking alone in the dark looking around the corners, just waiting for someone or something to pop out and attack. I never know what my attacker may be. It may be a tin can rolling in the street, a stray cat, or an armed and angry person set on hurting me. The threats can be minimal or extremely dangerous but I treat them all like a life-threatening experience.

There is no off switch on my trauma. I have taken tremendous strides at working on the after effects of such a traumatic event. I completely changed my diet, started focusing on myself, and now take the time to recognize when a stressful situation is happening. I also practice the techniques I learned over the past three years to promote calm and relaxation.

I want to emphasize the fact that not everything is awful. It does get better and every time I doubt myself, all I need to do is take a look at my son. Cole has come so far in the past three years. We are no longer in the thick of treatment with scary side effects and almost daily hospital visits. We are currently getting blood counts once a month and see the oncologist every two months. As things continue to go well and the oncologists distance themselves and the visits become farther apart, I get nervous, like a trapeze artist performing a spectacular routine high in the sky with no safety net below.

Reminding myself of the age old saying "no news is good news" and applying it to the longer time frame between visits means Cole is progressing. This is where my mantra comes into play. Take it "one day at a time". It gets to be too overwhelming when you look too far ahead, and the mind wanders to the "what ifs" and "this could happens". Living in the moment is very hard to do, but it's a blessing and it's beautiful when you can focus on the present and enjoy every single moment in life.

It does get easier after the bell is rung. Yes, there is the possibility for long-term side effects, but I continue to remind myself to focus on the now and bask in the glorious realm of survivorship.

One of my very good friends often reminds me of a phrase that she continues to use. I might call it her mantra. She often states "I get to…" as a prefix to something unpleasant or unexpected. As an example, two days ago we had an oncology appointment. This appointment comes less than a week before Cole's Make-A-Wish trip to Pearl Harbor. I'm already super anxious about the impending travel and flying across the country and then across the ocean to our island paradise. But pair that with a scheduled oncologist appointment and blood counts and I'm a bit of a mess. In Leila's world she would tell me to say, "I get to take Cole to his oncologist appointment in two days," reminding me that I am blessed to still have my son and still get to do these things that we may not want to do. It's a privilege to be here in this world, every single day. Saying "I get to" before doing something you think you "have" to do puts everything into perspective. We **get** to live this life and it's an honor.

Cole has now been out of treatment for seven months. Last week was the day he was actually supposed to end treatment - May 23, 2023. When that day came it felt surreal. So many things went through my mind. Did we make the right choice? Yes, I believe we made an informed decision along with Cole's doctors and years of research to back their opinions. I don't know what other side effects Cole would have suffered had we continued when it wasn't completely necessary.

What would the last seven months have looked like if we needed to continue treatment? Well, I don't want to entertain those thoughts because the after-treatment life is so much different than the in-treatment life. Yes, I say that there is still anxiety and sometimes it feels worse than when Cole was in treatment, but the anxiety is due to the traumatic experience of childhood cancer and its after effects, not solely due to the act of ending treatment.

I also look at Cole and how far he has come to ease my anxiety and fears. In May of last year, he had a life-threatening appendicitis and we spent over a week in the hospital. By the grace of God and an amazing surgeon's hands, my son is still with us today. May 2022, Cole weighed 20-25 pounds less than now due to not being able to eat after the surgery. Also, he couldn't walk for long, missed the last month of school, and certainly couldn't work out or lift weights. May 2023, Cole is in the gym five plus days a week, just completed his first high school combine, got a text from a college football coach today, is scheduled for two college courses for his senior year of high school and can certainly stand, walk, lift, and run.

Cole made amazing strides in the last seven months. Yes, he still has a long way to go, but, wow has he come far and I am so proud. For the past three years, I was in survival mode and crisis mode and switched between the two often. I was so used to expecting something dark and dangerous around the corner that I couldn't see the light shining from the stars illuminating my path. Good things do happen throughout treatment and better things happen when it ends. Not every day will be easy and yes, there will be trying times and bouts of anxiety, but follow the advice we received on the first day of diagnosis and don't look back, don' t look forward, just take it all "one day at a time".

Cole

When I rang the bell, my life changed for the better. When I was diagnosed, my life changed in a way I could never imagine. Everything was out of my control and my whole life revolved around my treatment. Every single aspect of my life linked back to treatment, and I was constantly reminded that I was no longer in control.

If I wanted to go hang out with my friends, I needed to wear a mask and be careful not to be exposed to germs. I couldn't go out and swim in creeks and lakes or even go to a public pool or water park. I couldn't do the one thing that I loved, which was play football. For three long seasons, I sat on the sideline and watched my friends play the game I loved.

Fast forward through all the treatments, hospital stays, pokes and prods and month after month of poison cocktails and spinal taps, in October of this past year, it all came to an end. I was finally free and able to get back to a normal life. Right after ending treatment, I felt a little difference but not much.

As the months went by, I got stronger and stronger and I was able to work out longer, lift heavier, and run faster. I started hanging out with my friends again and this summer is the first summer that I will be able to swim in public pools. In just a few short days, I will be in Hawaii relaxing on the beach and swimming in the ocean. I waited over three long years to do some of the things I loved before I was diagnosed. I can't wait to jump in the ocean, snorkel with sea turtles and go down the slide in the pool.

Another thing I am really looking forward to is my senior year of high school. I started high school on treatment, and next year I will graduate and be off to college. I can finally enjoy all the things in my life without my diagnosis and treatment controlling my life.

I want to tell those in the fight right now that it does get better. Sometimes it's really hard to imagine your life will ever be the same and it's not exactly the same, but it does return closer to normal. Sure, I still have doctor's appointments, crazy anxiety and other hardships, but it's nothing like it was during treatment and it gets better as time goes on. Keep going and keep pushing. There will be good days and bad days but as time goes on, there are way more good days than bad.

If you have been in the fight like I have, you can relate to everything I experienced in this book. I'm not going to lie, it was very hard for me to share all the deep, dark moments of my journey, but if it helps just one person, it was worth all the hours I spent remembering my story and writing it down to inspire someone else.

CHAPTER 15

An Amazing Journey

If you had just one wish after a particularly harrowing journey, what would you choose?

Laura

Our trip to Hawaii was a dream come true and the perfect example of paradise. For one full week, there were no worries, no fear, and no anxiety. For one week, we were just a family on an amazing journey to fill our souls and replenish our strength.

On June 5, 2023 we were able to take a trip to Hawaii as a family to realize Cole's wish to see Pearl Harbor. When we were first introduced to Make-A-Wish, Cole had absolutely no clue what he would choose when he was ready to experience his wish. Asking a teenager to pick one thing in the world that they would love to experience, no holds barred, literally puts the world at their fingertips.

In the beginning of treatment, before COVID, we knew a Make-A-Wish experience was on the table but we were told Cole had the option to wait until he was out of treatment to make travel safer if that's what he chose. So, Cole originally thought we would go to Europe and tour all of the World War II sites including sites in Germany, Italy, and/or Poland. As I mentioned before, Cole loves history and World War II is his favorite historical time period. Easy decision, right? Well when COVID unleashed its chaos on the world, Make-A-Wish and many other organizations and entities suspended travel. When travel was finally allowed once again (after the pandemic), international travel was not an option. We totally understood, but this meant Cole needed to go in a different direction for his wish.

Cole was still in treatment at the point travel was reinstated so he had time to decide his wish. It really wasn't an easy decision. At one point, he wanted to give back and start his own organization that connects pediatric cancer patients to their favorite sports teams by sending them fan gear, but there was little guidance on "philanthropic wishes" as they called them and starting a foundation is a huge undertaking.

So, we went back to square one. Our family urged Cole to do something for himself and really think of a wish that would make him happy. Understanding that we always strive to give back and starting a nonprofit organization is the ultimate goal for our family, he chose to visit Pearl Harbor. A United States site of World War II and in the exotic and tropical state of Hawaii; we couldn't think of anything he would enjoy more.

There was one tiny hump to jump over, however. The boys have never flown. My husband and I flew many times, but we haven't flown in years (at least since the boys were born). So, their first flight would be a non-stop 10-hour flight across the country. When we do things, we do them big.

Another detail to mention is a story involving my parents. My stepdad passed away from cancer on January 18, 2023. He was Cole's biggest support and cheered him on from the day he was diagnosed, even making him a sign for his end of treatment celebration because he was too sick to attend.

I mentioned he was a physician assistant and helped us give Cole his chemo shots at home. What I don't believed I mentioned, was that he switched careers and worked as a vaccine sales representative for a large pharmaceutical company for many years. His company often had conferences in different states and we were able to go to California and Florida a few times when I still lived at home. They also had several sales incentives, including trips to exotic locations. One year, the incentive was a single trip for the person with the most sales in a specific territory. The destination? Hawaii.

Knowing my mom is a huge *Hawaii Five -O* fan and always wanted to visit the Aloha state, he worked very hard to achieve the most sales possible. When the deadline came and the reward was given to the victor, he found out he came in second place. There would be no Hawaii trip for my parents.

So, when my stepdad got very sick and we were at my mom's house constantly, we were in the process of deciding Cole's wish. A few days before my stepdad passed, Cole chose Hawaii without any of us knowing the aforementioned story. The day my stepdad, or Pap-Paw, as the boys called him passed away our Make-A-Wish volunteer texted me that we were approved for the trip. We were going to Hawaii.

Not wanting to leave my mom alone and wanting her to come with us if possible, I mentioned the possibility of her coming along to see if she would be interested. She immediately said my stepdad must have had something to do with it and told me the story. Her decision was easy.

She was coming along. Even though Make-A-Wish did not include her as the wish family, she was able to come as a non-participant. This is kind of confusing, but basically, she was able to come along and enjoy the vacation with us if she paid for her trip.

So, on June 4th we packed all of our suitcases into my mom's SUV and drove to Newark, NJ in preparation for our early flight the next morning. I'm immediately reminded of two separate occasions on the night before a particularly stressful event, I was a bit of a mess. The experiences I'm referring to are the eve of my half marathon and the eve of Cole's bell ringing ceremony. I was filled with both nerves and excitement. It had been years since we traveled and maybe even longer since we had carefree relaxation in the company of family.

The morning of our flight, we arrived at the airport super early to make sure we were able to get our bags checked, get through security and find our gate without running through the airport like the McAllister family in *Home Alone*. Though things are definitely different in 2023, I really thought we resembled Kevin and his family racing franticly through the crowd filled area, suitcases in tow, scrambling to find the appropriate gate. Airports are confusing, some more than others, but we found our gate with plenty of time to spare.

When it was time to board the plane, the pilot approached me and asked if I was Cole's mom. Of course, I said yes and he explained that he knew we were going on a Make-A-Wish trip and wanted to know if the boys wanted to sit in the cock pit and meet the rest of the crew. Cole and

Kaden both looked at me and nodded so we were ushered onto the plane and into the cock pit. The pilots were so amazing and chatted with us a few minutes as the rest of the passengers boarded. Cole and Kaden sat in the special seats and we took the obligatory photos. United Airlines had the most amazing and thoughtful crew and I was incredibly grateful for our experience.

We were not seated together on the flight to Hawaii, although we were close. I sat next to the nicest couple and carried on a conversation with them throughout the trip. You will be amazed to know that this husband and wife were on their way to Hawaii because the husband, an employee of a pharmaceutical company, won the company's sale incentive trip. Of course, I told them our story. I firmly believe there are no coincidences and everything happens for a reason. I know my stepdad is smiling up in Heaven and happy we were all finally able to go to paradise together.

When we landed in Honolulu, we were all struck with the absolute beauty of Hawaii. Not only the beauty, but the kindness of everyone we encountered on our trip, made my soul happy. The Aloha spirit is alive and well in Hawaii and their culture is one full of love and kindness.

Make-A-Wish really thought of everything and we had an amazing experience. I want to share our trip with you for several reasons. If you are a family in the fight, know that each chapter varies and every wish is also different, but I hope by sharing our experience it may answer some questions and ease some fears. If you are a supporter and advocate for pediatric cancer patients, sharing our Make-A-Wish experience serves as an amazing example of a supportive organization and the importance to provide these types of supports to families. We have been through so much in the past three years and without Make-A-Wish, we would not have been able to take this trip. The kindness, support, care, and attention we received was more than I ever imagined and everything we absolutely needed.

Make-A-Wish provided a rental car for our family of five. We were driving in style in our white, Chrysler mini-van! It was actually amazing and very convenient. The resort was about 20 minutes from the airport and located in Kapolei, Hawaii. The Ko-Olina Beach Club was near the Disney resort, Aulani, and located in an absolutely beautiful area. The colors in Hawaii are absolutely gorgeous. This may seem odd, but the colors of the sky, water, grass, and just about everything are so vibrant and bold. Even our photos conveyed the beauty of the area which is usually difficult for me to do as I'm pretty unskilled at photography.

The day of our arrival, we spent time at the resort and got acclimated to our new residence for the next seven days. The time change didn't bother us too much on the way over, but we did go to bed at 7:30 PM that first night.

We received the itinerary with all the details of our trip including our boarding passes for the flights, rental car information, hotel reservation, and activity information with specific directions. The day of arrival and the following day were free, with our first activity occurring on Wednesday. Cole was given a list of possible activities and asked to rate his top four. Make-A-Wish would cover two activities (this varies by chapter). Cole was granted a private tour of Pearl Harbor and the USS Missouri as this was the ultimate goal of the trip and the Jurassic Park tour at Kualoa Ranch.

Wednesday was our first activity planned by Make-A-Wish and consisted of the Jurassic Park tour on the grounds where many of the movies were filmed. The location was about 30 minutes from the hotel and we were absolutely stunned by the beauty of the drive to the ranch. The flowers and trees were absolutely gorgeous and the scenery was not like anything we have ever seen.

When we got to the ranch, we were stunned even more by the beauty surrounding us at that moment. There is a reason so many movies and TV shows are filmed at this location. The natural beauty of the area is exquisite. As we sat and waited for the tour to begin, someone asked if someone named Cole was waiting for the tour. Cole raised his hand quietly and the nicest lady came over to him and gave him a special name tag and bag of souvenirs including a Jurassic Park T-shirt. I really can't keep track of the amount of times I cried on this trip, due to the absolute kindness of everyone, but I do know I cried a few times during the experience at the ranch.

Finally, the tour was about to start. The most vibrant tour guide approached us and got everyone together in a group. He explained everything that we would see and gave us instructions. The tour was given in a convertible bus type vehicle and we were warned many times it would be a bumpy ride.

For the next two hours, we explored the ranch with Koa, one of the nicest humans I've met. He stayed after the tour and spoke to our family, giving us the best tips and tricks and letting us know where we should go to find the best location to swim with sea turtles (my favorite). One thing that struck me was the ability of Koa to talk to each one of us, know all of our names in a short period of time, and create a bond with all of us. I got to know everyone on the tour, where they were from and what they did for a living. It was a great experience. We all had an amazing time.

Thursday was another free day and we took Koa's advice to walk to Paradise Cove near our resort and attempt to snorkel while seeing some sea turtles. Snorkeling is an art and there is a learning curve that had me swallowing salt water and shooting it out of my nose. Once I got the hang of it, I was amazed at the beautiful fish swimming amongst the coral and rocks just below my floating body. We all tried snorkeling and we were able to swim with a few sea turtles. It was an absolutely amazing experience and it didn't cost a thing (other than the cost of some masks and snorkels).

Spending time at the resort helped us refuel for the next experience on Friday, the reason for the trip. Pearl Harbor is absolutely breath-taking. I saw that same smile on my child's face when he rang the bell at the end of treatment reappear while he was exploring both Pearl Harbor and the USS Missouri. To say Cole was in his element, is an understatement. He was so excited, you could almost see the electricity running through his body.

When we arrived to Pearl Harbor bright and early on Friday morning, we were immediately taken aback by the absolute beauty and solemn nature of the site. Upon arrival, we checked in at the gift shop and awaited further instructions. While we waited, Cole was let loose in the gift/book shop and I could immediately see his excitement. In addition to history, Cole loves to read and has quite a collection of World War II related historical and historical fiction books on the dedicated bookshelf in his room.

I have a pretty good idea where Cole's love of history, reading, and endless pursuit of knowledge originated. Though there is a lot of debate regarding nature vs. nurture and if we are born with certain personality traits or if we learn them as a product of our environment, I believe genetics does have a role in certain elements of our personalities which, in turn, dictates the field of study we gravitate towards. My dad studied history/secondary education in college and is rarely seen without a book in close proximity.

My father's love of history and exploring events of the past found its way to me and ultimately to Cole. Military history and historical events related to World War II specifically runs through our veins and creates a passion urging us to learn more regarding events that occurred long before we were born. I tell you this to reiterate the significance of our visit to Pearl Harbor, something Cole waited years to see.

When Weston approached our family seated on the bench outside of the gift shop, I immediately knew he and Cole would become friends for the next couple of hours. If the Marvel lanyard hanging out of his pocket didn't indicate he was similar in nature to my son, it was absolutely evident in the way he spoke about all the events surrounding the attack on Pearl Harbor. As we made our way through the museums, I looked over at Cole a few times and could actually see him soaking in all the knowledge like a sponge holding the maximum amount of water possible, trying to squeeze in every molecule. An instant connection was made between Cole and our private guide/personal historian as he asked many questions and held a conversation with Weston throughout our time together.

For the next few hours, we explored the grounds of Pearl Harbor eventually making our way to the USS Arizona memorial where we walked directly above the tomb of countless soldiers trapped in the water below. The area was sacred, calm, quiet and the experience of seeing it first hand is extremely impactful and emotional.

Saying goodbye to Weston was difficult but we are extremely grateful for the experience. To say he had an impact on our family is an understatement. After our time with Weston, Cole, still radiating electricity and sparkle from every ounce of his being, pulled me aside and gently spoke into my ear. The words Cole spoke immediately brought a smile to my face. He said "Mom, I know what I want to do now. I want to do this. I want to be a historian and share my knowledge with other people."

Preparing for college and the questions that come along with choosing a major have been a contentious journey. Just as the wish process was difficult and then all of a sudden, one day it clicked and then a few short months later we were at Pearl Harbor, the choice of a major and future career path hasn't always been clear. Until now. Thanks to Weston and the experience of immersing my son in military history for a day, Cole now knows he would like to hold a similar position.

As I allow myself a momentary glimpse into the future, I can see Cole with his group sharing all his knowledge as he guides them on the exploration of a historical site. The experience of that day brings me back to a phrase I hear often. "Always be yourself, you never know who you are inspiring." I'm guessing Weston didn't know he would inspire a pediatric cancer survivor from Pennsylvania that day, but because he was his true, authentic self, he propelled my son to decide something in the future.

The future. For a pediatric cancer family, it can be a scary concept. We don't know what the future brings and when in the throes of trauma, we can't even begin to look forward. The whole purpose of this book, sharing our journey with the world, and describing an amazing celebration at the end of treatment is to make the future brighter for someone else.

Our mantra throughout this journey has always been "one day at a time". Yes, live in the present, be grateful for every experience and every moment, don't look back, don't look forward and live "one day at a time" UNTIL you are able to get to the point in your journey when you glimpse into the future and allow yourself to be inspired, making a decision that will propel you into the after-cancer experience. No, you won't forget the journey, but hopefully the trauma will ease and your mind will clear just enough to take a peak into the future and see nothing but rainbows and sunshine, inspired by a positive experience and a magical wish.

EPILOGUE

Cole and I hope that we were inspirational guides throughout the story of our journey and inspired you to continue in your journey whatever that may be. We share a few thoughts and feelings regarding the experience of making a private journey public in the hopes to inspire, advocate, and propel change.

How is it possible to believe in something without seeing it for yourself? The answer is a simple but, powerful word: *faith*. Have faith in the unseen.

Sometimes it's incredibly hard for me to have faith that I am living according to God's word and taking the path He made for me to follow. I'm human. Not only am I human, but I feel like a mess of a human. I yell, I have a short temper, I hate my body, I can't think straight, and the anxiety well that's enough information for an entire book in and of itself. I compare myself to everything and everyone. Have you ever heard of the saying "comparison is the thief of joy?"

Well, I can attest that it is indeed true. I can never have joy in my accomplishments because I'm always comparing them to someone else's accomplishments and denouncing my triumphs as failures. How can I ever be happy in and with my own life when I am constantly comparing myself to someone totally different with different life experiences and accomplishments? Why are they better than me? Why is their experience more valid? The easy and truthful answer is this: they are not better. Their accomplishments are not more than what I am doing. Their experiences are not more valid than our family's experiences. However, they are different. Do not compare yourself to someone else because they are not you. Did you ever hear the saying: "the only person who can live your life is you". Well, it's completely true. Every experience you have, every accomplishment you make, and every day you are blessed to live on this Earth is amazing.

I am constantly telling myself lies when I compare what someone else is doing to myself and saying that my accomplishments are less than what they have done. It's so easy to see the grass on the other side of the fence and admire the lush and dense blades that are the brightest and thickest green you have ever seen. The grass is so amazing that you are no longer content observing it from the distance, but you need to get closer. So, you take the steps, two at a time, to lessen the distance and finally get to see the coveted grass up close and personal. When you get next to perfection, you realize it's not perfection at all. There are bare spots, frayed blades, and brown discoloration throughout.

It's so easy to look at someone's life and deem it as perfect from the outside until you get up close and personal and realize it's not perfect at all. Why? Because life isn't perfect, and we are all human. Give yourself grace, stop comparing your journey to someone else's experiences and tell that thief, comparison, to go take a hike. When you truly learn to live life by the moment and take every triumph and accomplishment by stride, celebrating the amazing opportunities life throws your way, then true happiness lies around the corner.

Is happiness perfect? No, it's not. I think that is why I struggle to truly be happy because when something goes sideways, I immediately turn in the towel and say "well, there it goes. Happiness is gone." It is possible to be happy when things are not perfect.

Bob Cratchit had a tough life. He was poor, barely had enough money to feed his family and put a roof over their heads. His son was very sick and there was a lot of uncertainty in his future. Oh, and we can't forget he had pretty much the worst boss ever. But, you know what? I am immediately drawn to scenes when he is with his family and smiling, enjoying every single moment of his imperfect life.

Happiness in the imperfection can also be found on the pediatric cancer floor or clinic. If an outsider walks onto the floor, they may expect sullen room upon sullen room with children in an immense amount of pain and worried family members strewn about. No, this floor is not perfect in any sense of the word. Cancer should not happen, especially to our children. There is pain, there is sadness and there is trauma and lots of it. But, there is also joy and happiness in the imperfection.

Pediatric cancer patients have a glow and radiance about them like angels on Earth. They still smile and keep moving, "one day at a time", in the imperfection, pain, sadness and downright cruel reality of life at that moment. Because, at that moment there is no comparison to a "perfect life; there is joy in the "imperfect life".

Living in our lives of sorrow and imperfection without comparing them to others and wishing things were different is downright difficult.

However, when we are truly able to live "one day at a time" without looking to the past, future, or the seemingly perfect lawn across the street we can live in the moment and see the joy that exists right in that imperfect moment.

What do you say to someone whose child was just diagnosed with cancer? There are no words able to patch the hole the trauma that a childhood cancer diagnosis causes to parents' hearts.

In the same realm…what do you say to a teenager who was just diagnosed with cancer? A teenager who should be exploring life, learning and developing into a young adult and laying the foundation for the rest of their lives. Again, I can't think of anything that could be said to lessen the pain.

The pain of a cancer diagnosis will be in varying degrees. A teen diagnosed with cancer will need to face months or years of treatment with day after day of painful pokes and unpleasant chemo. If the teen is lucky, they will stay out of the hospital and endure most of these treatments in a clinic, but that is not always possible. Hospitalization away from friends and the disappointment of being left out of normal activities are all too common.

In our experience, there are no words to patch the pain. For those of us on the journey of pediatric cancer, other warriors and survivors who stand on the battle lines with us, organizations dedicated to supporting cancer fighters and their families, brave souls not scared away by the trauma and heartache and others who hold our hands and charge forward by our sides do not need to utter words.

Support, understanding, and the passion to fight are actions that speak louder than anything uttered from their lips.

We hope our heartbreaking, traumatic, vile, inspiring and sometimes comical story took you through the gamut of emotions as nothing is black and white in cancer, and there are varying degrees of gray with some brilliant colors of inspiring and beautiful moments sprinkled in between.

Sharing our story is not easy and was done with two distinct purposes. The first being a guiding light and hope in the tunnel of darkness for parents, caregivers, and fighters. You are not alone and never will be. We have been on this journey and understand it all too well. We hope that our words wrap you in an embrace and give you the strength to keep going, "one day at a time".

The second and different purpose of our story is propelling change. By sharing our experience, we hope to clear the path making the journey smoother for those who come after us. Increased support for the teenage population, better resources in smaller hospitals, the extinction of drug shortages, awareness, and advocating for better and safer treatments are all things that are needed. Step up and make a difference in future patients' experiences. Use our words to fuel your advocacy for pediatric cancer patients and take every step "one day at a time."

Printed in the USA
CPSIA information can be obtained
at www.ICGtesting.com
LVHW091201160923
758175LV00002B/201